BEWARE OF YOUR DOCTOR:
How to Survive the Medical System

Kfir Luzzatto, Ph.D., Dip. Hyp.

PINE 10

Pine Ten, LLC
205 N Michigan Ave.
Chicago, IL 60601

Fist publication, October 2018

ISBN: 978-1-938212-79-6

Table of Contents

Introduction

You know those pills that your doctor prescribed for you? There is at least a 20% chance that you don't need them and that they may be harming you.

I'm not pulling your leg. A research published in September 2017[1] found that on average in the United States 20.6% of overall medical care was unnecessary, including 22% of prescription medication. And if that was not enough, another study[2] found that 10–15% of diagnoses are wrong. Shocking, isn't it?

So if you have been conditioned to think that your doctor must be right and that you need to follow his or her prescription blindly, think again. Your health depends on your willingness to inquire, question, check, and double check, and on an understanding of the many possible pitfalls of the medical system. I cannot give you the strength and the willpower to question your doctor's recommendations, but I can give you the information you need to understand why you must question it. Moreover, I can certainly try to make it compelling for you to

---

[1] https://doi.org/10.1371/journal.pone.0181970
[2] https://qualitysafety.bmj.com/content/22/Suppl_2/ii21

ask yourself questions that may have a direct impact on the type and quality of the medical service to which you will have access, and to take an unbiased firsthand look at your situation. That is the purpose of this book.

If you have received a diagnosis of any kind, there are at least three questions that you must pose to yourself:

1. Does the diagnosis "feel" right to me?

2. Is my condition a widespread one right now?

3. Is the proposed treatment going to have a substantial impact on my life?

In the following chapters we will discuss these three questions in detail, as well as other more specific ones, including how to answer them and the meaning of the answer that you will give to them; but first we must understand why we need to question our doctor's diagnosis at all.

This book may be particularly helpful to people diagnosed with conditions of low or medium severity, because with very severe conditions most people will almost always seek a second and often a third opinion, thus substantially increasing the chances—but far from insuring—that the answer they will get in the end, is correct. But even if your diagnosis is that of a life-threatening condition, you may find some useful, thought-provoking information between these pages.

Most people will take a diagnosis of a common, not immediately life-threatening condition, at face value, particularly if it comes from a physician they have been seeing for a long time and never had complaints about, and even more so if it somehow fits with other perceived parameters such as age and medical history. Thus, many people will end up taking statins to lower their cholesterol, or beta blockers to deal with a suddenly discovered high blood pressure, simply on their physician's say-so, without questioning or probing his or her directives.[3] And in some cases (perhaps in many cases, as we will discuss in later chapters), the treatment will be unnecessary and its side effects could have been avoided.

Why have I written this book?

This book is based on facts and experiences, some related to my work and to information I have gathered over the years working on medical subjects, and others related to personal experience, mine and that of people close to me. I am a chemical engineer, a patent attorney, an inventor, and a writer (not necessarily in that order) and, as such, I enjoy a broad vision of many fields. This is particularly true because I have been working closely on medical subjects for many more years than I care to remember, and have absorbed a vast body of information. As a result, I have come to the realization that too many diagnoses result in unnecessary and harmful treatments, which can be avoided if the patient is aware of a few simple facts and is able to make his own enquiries before initiating treatment. The information needed to obtain a better and more appropriate treatment is not secret—it is available to everybody who wishes to take the time to read, compile, interpret, and draw conclusions from it. However, a synthetic treatment of this information is not readily available to the layperson, so since putting sometimes complicated facts into clear, easy-to-follow written form is what I do, I have made it my task to compile it. I am not adding any personal belief or coming up with any new theories of my own (and who would I be to do that). All I'm doing is taking the information that is hiding in plain sight and connecting the dots for you, my reader.

The purpose of this book is to provide eye-opening information written for the general public, without obfuscating

---

[3] From this point on I use the masculine for simplicity and to avoid the unhelpful repetition of "his or her" and "she or he," but everything should be taken to relate equally to male and female physicians and patients.

medical jargon, which will help the reader to navigate the maze of decisions that he has to make as a patient in the present-day medical system.

It so happens that if you want to get the medical treatment that you deserve, you must be assertive and knowledgeable. If you close your eyes and let the wind take you whichever direction it's blowing, there is no telling where you will wind up. So let's turn the page and start to navigate the puzzle using the knowledge that is out there for us to grasp.

CHAPTER 1
The Medical System and You

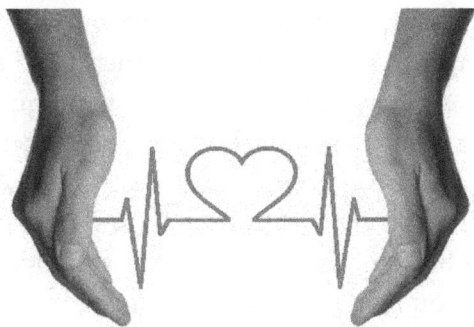

Successes and Failures of Modern Medicine

Modern medicine is simultaneously a tremendous success, and an utter failure. There is no denying that medical science has brought us almost magic treatments that save lives and improve the quality of life for entire patient populations that only a few decades ago were left untreated. Modern medicine can save you when you are in a critical condition, such as resulting from a car accident, a swiftly diagnosed brain hemorrhage, or an acute infection. My great aunt died of tuberculosis because antibiotics had not yet been invented, and my uncle died of a heart attack because at the time coronary bypasses were still considered an experimental procedure. The solution to those and many other illnesses have been largely found, but, on the way to producing those results, our individuality has been lost. We have become part of a range of statistics.

Human and mice both share about 97.5% of total working DNA (some articles give slightly different figures, but we won't split hairs here), and yet, we are so different. Rats live three years and we live (hopefully) 80–100 years. Those huge differences come from a mere 2.5% difference in DNA. Humans, in contrast, differ from one another in about 1% of the DNA. That may seem a small difference, but it is in fact huge in many senses. For instance, recent studies have shown that dietary advice is largely nonsensical, because some people will gain weight with the same diet that works wonders on others,[4] and the reason is that we are different. Each one of us is unique and reacts differently to different stimuli, be they foods or drugs. But that doesn't stop modern medicine from classifying us. According to your doctor, if you are a male, over 50, and have condition X, you need the blue pill, and if you are a woman over 65 who has condition Y, you need the pink one. But two men over 50 with the same condition will react differently to their pill, and so will two women over 65.

A paper[5] published by scientists at the Weizmann Institute recently highlighted these differences. It demonstrated statistically significant interpersonal variability in the glycemic response to different bread types, suggesting that the lack of phenotypic difference between the bread types stems from a person-specific effect—or, translated into understandable, simple English: each person reacts individually to the type of

---

[4] https://www.nytimes.com/2016/12/12/health/weight-loss-obesity.html?mcubz=2

[5] http://www.cell.com/cell-metabolism/abstract/S1550-4131(17)30288-7

bread. It further concluded that a crossover trial showed no differential clinical effect of white versus sourdough bread and that the glycemic response to the two types of bread varies greatly across people. So, when the various health authorities and organizations tell you that whole grain is good for your health and is better for you than something else if your blood sugar level is elevated, they don't know what they are talking about. It is understandable that they feel a need to say something, to give some guidance. However, instead of stating nonsense, they would do better simply by telling you that which kind of food is good for you cannot be predicted, and that you should learn what's best for you on your own. Oh, but then that wouldn't be *real* guidance, would it? It would undermine their authority, wouldn't it?

They Don't Believe in Us
The underlying assumption of the medical system, gently put, is that we don't have the willpower—let alone the ability—to help ourselves and, besides, that we don't need to. The doctors know best and we shouldn't get in their way. We cannot be relied on to do the right thing, and since it can be done for us, it would be irresponsible to leave it to us. This paternalistic approach to our health has turned us into useless and passive individuals. But it wasn't always like that.[6] In the past, much of the work was left to the patient and to his family, simply because they didn't have easy access to medical treatment. Still, the conviction with which medical doctors have looked down upon their patients and have prescribed wrong cures is not new. As a result, people have tried for ages to cure themselves with remedies that were downright dangerous. For instance, today it is obvious to us that the idea that leeches had the potential to

---

[6] More about that in Chapter 3.

cure severe infections was sheer madness, but at the time the average physician considered it a completely reasonable approach. On the other hand, some old home remedies make sense even today.[7]

The accumulation of knowledge in the medical field should have benefited us by substantially increasing the ability of the patient to help himself, whenever possible, and to rely on medical treatment only when the problem was beyond the reach of the individual's more limited knowledge. But on the contrary, we have become lazy and have lost the will to help ourselves. We have been conditioned to look elsewhere for the quick fix.

Why practice physical therapy at home to fix a painful hip or knee, enduring pain and working hard for a long period of time (and possibly failing), when we can get a shiny new cobalt-chrome one installed into us while we sleep? And why should we go to the pain of exercising and reducing our caloric intake, giving up that creamy stuff that we really like, while we can get bariatric surgery (stomach resizing) if we can't control our cravings?

But even without going to the extremes of surgery, we have been conditioned to reach for a pill for pretty much everything. If we can't sleep, we don't ask ourselves if we are doing something bad to our circadian rhythm (like, for instance, working at our PC just before bedtime) and what changes we should make to our routine to fix it; we take sleeping pills. If our lower back aches, we don't ask ourselves if we are sitting wrong, or too much, and what we should do to make it stop; we take a painkiller.

It is not our fault (well, in fact it is, but we can claim extenuating circumstances)—that is what our world looks like,

---

[7] https://www.rd.com/health/wellness/old-time-home-remedies

what we have been brought up to believe, and what we see everybody else doing.

But now it's time to wake up and look beyond the tip of our nose for solutions that are out there, over which we may have at least some measure of control.

Reasons for the Scary Numbers

Once upon a time, there was a thing called "bedside manner." I still remember our family physician, who, when I was a little boy, used to come to our house when I was sick. He always sat with me on my bed, asked questions, and then sat with my parents for a cup of coffee. I felt that he *knew* me and I trusted him to give me the medicine I needed. When he said that whatever illness I had would pass in a couple of days, I felt better already because he had followed me since I was a baby and knew how I would respond to his treatment or to my mother's chicken soup. But those days are past and gone. Today's physicians must treat so many people in so little time that they simply cannot get to know you. And then, they have the cursed thing called the "protocol," which they must follow, or they may be accused of malpractice.

The other curse of modern medicine is specialization. If your little finger hurts, you must go and see a Little Finger Specialist to whom your general practitioner will refer you. He knows everything about little fingers, but he doesn't know you. To him you are not a person with all the complexity that it involves, you are a "hurting little finger case" to be treated according to protocol.

As reported above, a recent study in the US[8] found that 20.6% of overall medical care was unnecessary, including 22% of prescription medication. And if that was not enough, another

---

[8] https://doi.org/10.1371/journal.pone.0181970

study[9] found that 10–15% of diagnoses are wrong. That means that if your doctor prescribed a drug for you, in 22% of the cases you are taking something you don't need. For instance, let's assume that you were prescribed a COX-2 inhibitor, which is a common and effective nonsteroidal anti-inflammatory drug (NSAID) used for the relief of pain, fever, swelling, and tenderness caused by arthritis, as well as for acute pain and menstrual cramps— truly a "life saver" if you are in pain. If you really need it, then you must make peace with the negative effects that it potentially carries with it. But if you don't need it, you may be exposing yourself to a host of severe side effects, such as serious stomach and intestinal ulcers, for no reason. If your doctor was wrong in his prescription and you are one of the 22 patients in 100 who do not need the drug and to whom the drug is not going to do any good, the following are some of the side effects that you may experience (the actual list is longer):

• chest pain, weakness, shortness of breath, slurred speech, problems with vision or balance;

• black, bloody, or tarry stools;

• coughing up blood or vomit that looks like coffee grounds;

• swelling or rapid weight gain;

• urinating less than usual or not at all;

• nausea, upper stomach pain, itching, loss of appetite, dark urine, clay-colored stools, jaundice (yellowing of the skin or eyes);

• skin rash, bruising, severe tingling, numbness, pain, muscle weakness; or

• severe skin reaction—fever, sore throat, swelling in your face or tongue, burning in your eyes, skin pain, followed by a

---

[9] https://qualitysafety.bmj.com/content/22/Suppl_2/ii21

red or purple skin rash that spreads (especially in the face or upper body) and causes blistering and peeling.

"Side effect" is a laundered term for "harmful result of taking a drug." If you have no choice and must take the drug because of your condition, then it makes sense to brave the side effects, but are you willing to chance them for nothing? Of course you are not. That is why you need to go on reading.

Why Do Doctors Make Mistakes?
This question was analyzed in a 2014 research report,[10] which concluded that *"Cognitive errors made by doctors while diagnosing cases form a substantial part of preventable mistakes. Research has shown that cognitive errors are often a result of faulty reasoning rather than a lack of knowledge."* This conclusion is in line with another review by Pat Croskerry, published in 2013,[11] which states that *"Diagnostic error has multiple causes, but principal among them are cognitive errors. Usually, it's not a lack of knowledge that leads to failure, but problems with the clinician's thinking ... common illnesses are commonly misdiagnosed. For example, physicians know the pathophysiology of pulmonary embolus in excruciating detail, yet because its signs and symptoms are notoriously variable and overlap with those of numerous other diseases, this important diagnosis was missed a staggering 55% of the time in a series of fatal cases."* **Fifty-five percent of the time!**

My mother-in-law always placed unreserved faith in her doctor because he was "a professor." Any attempts to convince her that his diagnoses had to be viewed with a critical eye were doomed to failure, because he was so "knowledgeable."

---

[10] https://journals.lww.com/academicmedicine/fulltext/2014/01000/
Why_ Do_Doctors_Make_Mistakes__A_Study_of_the_Role.31.aspx
[11] http://www.uphs.upenn.edu/gme/pdfs/Croskerry_Mindfulenss
%20to%20Mindful%20practice_NEJM.pdf

Knowledge (or lack thereof), however, doesn't play a big part in the problem.

A greater understanding of this topic is found in a fascinating book by Nobel Prize Laureate Daniel Kahneman,[12] in which the faulty intuition mechanism is elucidated. The mechanism is explained by the action of two systems, System 1 and System 2.[13] According to Kahneman, *"System 1 operates automatically and quickly, with little or no effort and no sense of voluntary control. System 2 allocates attention to the effortful mental activities that demand it, including complex computations. The operations of System 2 are often associated with the subjective experience of agency, choice, and concentration."* So what happens when a doctor is presented with information regarding a patient and makes a wrong diagnosis? According to Kahneman's explanation: *"When an incorrect intuitive judgment is made, System 1 and System 2 should both be indicted. System 1 suggested the incorrect intuition, and System 2 endorsed it and expressed it in a judgment. However, there are two possible reasons for the failure of System 2—ignorance or laziness."*

Ignorance certainly plays a part in it, and I will give examples later in this book, but at the cost of sounding harsh, I will concentrate more on the issue of "laziness." The reason is clear: if your doctor is ignorant, no amount of industriousness will help. On the contrary, on occasions ignorant but industrious doctors may do much more harm than lazy ones. But "laziness," in the context of Kahneman's teachings, should not be taken as a conscious unwillingness of your doctor to make an effort to reach the correct diagnosis or to prescribe the correct cure. Conversely, in almost every case he will believe that

---

[12] Kahneman, Daniel. *Thinking, Fast and Slow.*
[13] These two systems are called by Croskerry and other researchers Type 1 and Type 2 processes.

he is doing a magnificent job, but he will trip over the mechanism of his System 1 and System 2 behavior for a number of reasons, not least among them the damnable protocols and the lack of time that he has to invest in each patient. They will be a cause of the gullibility of System 2, which will then believe the intuitive, easy, and wrong solution offered by System 1.

There is obviously more to it than this rather simplistic explanation, and a study of Kahneman's book may provide those interested in a deeper understanding of the process with a much broader perspective, but this brief explanation is sufficient for the purpose of this discussion. Another important aspect of the problem is likely to be connected with the essence of intuitive heuristics: when faced with a difficult question, we often answer an easier one instead, usually without noticing the substitution. In other words, when answering the question "could the symptoms mean that the patient has this uncommon condition" requires substantial effort, while the question "could this be a common cold" is an easy one to answer, the wrong diagnosis of "common cold" is likely to result.[14]

The God Complex
Not all doctors have a God complex, but I have met a few who do. Those are the ones who will look at you with condescension when you make a suggestion, such as perhaps taking another test or considering an alternative treatment. The ones who resist suggestions from their patients are also those who are less likely to doubt their own conclusions, no matter how faulty they may be. I have made it a practice, whenever I meet one of those God-like doctors, to run the other way. Of course, you may run the risk of falling into the hands of one of those when you are more

---

[14] This could also be the reason behind the missed diagnosis of pulmonary embolus mentioned by Croskerry.

vulnerable, such as if you have been hospitalized and are at the mercy of the system. You must still find the strength to question, inquire, and doubt, because the chances of becoming the victim of a hospital mistake are not negligible. At the cost of sounding like an alarmist, I will cite a 2013 article that investigates the harm caused to American patients, which is associated with hospital care.[15] This review estimates the number of premature deaths associated with preventable harm to patients at more than 400,000 per year. It further indicates that serious harm seems to be 10- to 20-fold more common than lethal harm (or in other words, 4 to 8 million!).

That's why I find Dr. Ken Berry's statement: *"Doctors became distracted and disenchanted, stopped paying attention, and worse, stopped caring"* in his book,[16] both courageous and inspiring. You won't find many practicing physicians who are ready to come out publicly and state this simple truth. I know that many practicing physicians—possibly the vast majority of them—are caring people who want to give their patients the best possible treatment, but this will not happen until the medical profession recognizes its shortcomings.

The Great Doctors

I wouldn't be doing justice to the subject if I failed to say a few words about the great doctors. I have met many caring, passionate, empathic doctors, and a few who are true angels of mercy. I have felt how talking to some of them really lifted my spirit and restored (albeit, temporarily) my belief in the medical system. Others have made miracles or, at least, have done everything to make miracles possible, regardless of the actual outcome.

---

[15] https://www.ncbi.nlm.nih.gov/pubmed/23860193
[16] Berry MD, Ken D. *Lies My Doctor Told Me: Medical Myths That Can Harm Your Health.*

It may even be that this description is true for most physicians. But even the best, most caring doctors make mistakes. Some mistakes can be the result of the system in which they work, the long hours, the facilities available to them, and sometimes even a result of their eagerness to go the extra mile for their patient. Statistically, they may be great, but we must always remember that **we are not statistics—we are persons**. A doctor with a 99.9% success rate means nothing to us, if we are the one patient in 1,000 whom he failed. And if he has a history of solving our own problems brilliantly in the past, that doesn't mean that he will not fail us this time. Even if we love, respect, or revere him, and even if he's our friend from kindergarten or a blood relative, it is still our responsibility to check on him every step of the way, to make sure that we are getting what we need. And we will have only ourselves to blame if we fail to do so.

Takeaways from This Chapter:

▶ We are all different, and a broadly accepted therapy that works well for others may not be right for you.
▶ We have been conditioned to look for "easy" solutions, reaching out for a pill almost immediately instead of trying to find out if *we* can do something to help ourselves.
▶ If more than 20% of overall medical care administered is unnecessary (including 22% of prescription medication), it is very possible that you are exposing yourself to undesirable side effects to no useful end.
▶ Physicians make mistakes for a variety of reasons and a substantial part of preventable mistakes is due to cognitive errors.

CHAPTER 2
Too Old to Live

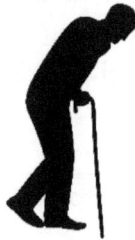

My urge to write this book has its roots in my earliest encounter with a manifestation of pernicious medical malpractice, some thirty years ago. My father was 73 years old at the time, in good shape but with a strong penchant for chocolate that may have been the reason for his clogged arteries. He had suddenly experienced chest pain, which an EKG had easily diagnosed to be a bad case of atherosclerosis. The seriousness of his condition, however, required an angioscopy to determine. Obviously worried, I made inquiries that led me to a professor, who was considered the leading cardiologist in the country and the most dexterous performer of angioscopy ever. Luckily enough, an acquaintance of mine worked as his assistant, and we were able to schedule the procedure quickly.

As soon as the angioscopy ended the professor called me aside and this is what he told me:

"I'm afraid there is little that we can do for your father. He has a 90% occlusion of the main artery. Considering his age and condition, he won't be able to withstand surgery. But don't worry—we will give him medication that will help him enjoy a reasonable quality of life."

"For how long?" I asked.

"Oh, at least for a few months," he said casually.

Even then, as he was dealing this blow to me, I couldn't help noticing how smug he was in his self-importance, with the countenance of a man who holds the power of life and death over mere mortals.

"Give me the film of the angioscopy," I said, "and we'll be on our way."

He sent me the film with his assistant, who tried in vain to convince me to listen to his boss and to let my father die peacefully, without attempting to subject him to uselessly painful procedures. I took the film, collected my father, and left.

To cut a long story short, my father lived to see 97. He had coronary bypass surgery done twice (a lousy surgeon botched the first one), as well as a replacement of the mitral valve, which he had done at age 84. He was in relatively good health until a couple of years before his death.

The thought that this incompetent physician could have robbed my father of 24 years of his life has haunted me ever since. I have often wondered how many people whose only sin was their age this professor had sentenced to death in that offhand way of his, only because they didn't have someone like me, who was cheeky enough to challenge the diagnosis of a man who, in those days, was considered almost the emissary of God on Earth.

If this book has a mission, this is it: **Don't you ever allow a doctor to discourage you from doing what it takes to get well, no matter how great he and his milieu think he is.**

Ageism

Ageism or age bias or discrimination, is not a new concept. It was identified and discussed a long time ago. One review[17] concludes that *"Despite the slightly higher risks of perioperative mortality and morbidity in older people, if they are selected appropriately they are likely to gain substantial health benefits from cardiological interventions."* However, surgeons who are sensitive about their success rate will sometimes refuse to operate on older patients because of such "slightly higher risk."

Such discriminatory practices may have legal implications, when a patient is denied treatment solely on account of his or her age. A discussion of the legal implications can be found in an article in the *Marquette Elder's Advisor*.[18]

Dealing with ageism is not simple, because the treating or referring physician may put forward a host of reasons, real or fictitious, why a given treatment should not be administered to a certain patient, or why he will not be able to survive surgery. He may or may not be right, but what is certain is that he is not automatically right. A study[19] carried out in Ireland in 2002 found both age and gender bias in the prescription of important secondary preventive therapies in primary care that may lead to

---

[17] Ageism in cardiology -
https://www.ncbi.nlm.nih.gov/pmc/articles/PMC1117086
[18] Age Discrimination in the Delivery of Health Care Services to Our Elders
- http://scholarship.law.marquette.edu/elders/vol11/iss1/3
[19] https://bpspubs.onlinelibrary.wiley.com/doi/pdf/10.1046/j.1365-2125.2003.01795.x

increased mortality from ischemic heart disease in these groups. In this study women were less likely to receive important preventive therapies than men.

But ageism does not stop there. Sometimes elder people may be more difficult to talk to, particularly if they are unwell or if their mind is not as sharp as it used to be, and physicians need a good supply of empathy and patience to deal with them. A busy doctor with no patience may reach a wrong conclusion about his patient's conditions, simply because he does not take the time to talk to him, and may prescribe a wrong (or no) therapy as a result. He may also feel that because of the patient's old age he cannot be expected to get much better anyway, and may allow himself to be less concerned about the prospect that his patient may die. All this may happen at an unconscious level, if the physician is a decent person, or at a conscious level if he is anything like my father's cardiologist and has a God complex. That's why if you accompany an elder person who is seeking medical assistance, you must be aware of this possible additional ageism effect and act as his surrogate in probing the diagnosis and the treatment he is receiving.

Other Forms of Bias

Ageism is not the only form of bias. Bias exists in many instances, not only with respect to surgical procedures, in which other aspects (such as a surgeon's reputation for success) may play a role, but in many and perhaps in all forms of medical treatment. However, because surgery often has to be performed without delay, a bias that causes a delay in the patient reaching a surgeon who is willing to perform the procedure may in itself be deleterious or cause him to reach a point in time when surgery can no longer be performed.

A review of the bias related to surgical procedures[20] (which the authors compassionately call "unconscious bias") concluded that *"Gender, race, and ethnicity are just a few potential stereotypes that may trigger unconscious bias in medical decisions."* Moreover, the authors conclude that *"Embracing a patient's sociocultural context requires empathy. Empathy is a powerful tool against unconscious bias … Unfortunately, surgeons are not at the top of the scale when compared with other specialists on a validated empathy scale, which may be influenced by the rigors of their training and job."*

A lack of empathy is what makes a physician tell a patient that he is too old to undergo a procedure, even when the clear outcome of withholding surgery means certain early death. Of course, this lack of empathy is wrapped up in confusing medical terms, but the net result it has is to discourage the patient from fighting for his life.

Students of the Bible know the passage in Numbers 22, where (in free translation) Balaam "came to curse the sons of Israel and found himself blessing them." This is somewhat similar to what organizations such as SurgeonRatings.Org[21] are doing, only in reverse. They mean well and in many cases may be doing well, but in other aspects they may unwittingly be exacerbating the problem. This is what its website states:

"To help you choose the best surgeon, our website tells you which doctors had relatively few deaths and other bad outcomes (based on our researchers' analysis of the data we had, including adjustments for the characteristics of the surgeons' patients) for 12 board categories of surgery, which doctors were most often recommended by other doctors, which hospitals used by the doctors had the best surgical outcomes, and other key facts, such as board certification, education, and training."

---

[20] https://www.ncbi.nlm.nih.gov/pmc/articles/PMC3417145
[21] http://www.checkbook.org/surgeonratings/

All true and correct but consider these two examples:

Surgeon A is very famous and makes tons of money in private practice, thanks to a very high success rate (and an extremely low mortality rate), due in part to a careful selection of patients. Old patients or those in poor physical conditions are rejected by him.

Surgeon B works in a hospital. He is very motivated and has made it his life mission to place his skills at the service of whoever needs them. As a result, he is completely unbiased in his choice of patients. He operates as long as there is a chance of saving the patient, regardless of age, physical condition, and any other consideration.

So who do you think will rate higher with SurgeonRatings.Org? Obviously it will be Surgeon A. That does not mean that both surgeons wouldn't be equally successful with the same patient. It does mean, however, that the public rating will increase the chances of a patient to be rejected by Surgeon A, whenever he thinks that the patient may ruin his statistics. He doesn't have a problem doing that, since the demand for successful surgeons is always greater than the supply.

The above does not imply that information like that supplied by SurgeonRating.Org is not useful. It is, because it reflects a statistical reality and provides a baseline for a patient to increase his chances. That information will be skewed, however, because it will glorify the less empathic surgeon and may downrate good ones for reasons over which they have no control, including a likely mortality or complications due to sanitary conditions at the hospital or at home. Accordingly, patients would be wise to cross-reference that information with other factors, some of which will be discussed in Chapter 11.

Allocation of Medical Resources

Sometimes you may have to fight for your life (or in less life-threatening cases, for your health), because the system makes decisions on allocating medical resources, which are always limited, according to rules that may be bendable. An extreme example is given in an article reviewing how the issue is handled in Switzerland,[22] and refers to the allocation of donor organs.

"In Switzerland, the Regulation on the Allocation of Organs for Transplantation (Regulation 810.212.4; enacted 16 March 2007; version of 1 May 2016) governs the allocation of the following donor organs: heart, lung, liver, kidney, pancreas, small intestine. Allocation rules are based on multiple criteria and differ (slightly) for different organs. In summary,

medical urgency: first priority is given to patients whose life would be at immediate risk if they would not receive the organ;
medical benefit: second priority is given to patients, for whom the greatest medical benefit is expected."

All fair and square, except, who makes the decision on who is the patient who may expect the greatest medical benefit? That is where the rule becomes somewhat flexible, because it is a matter of judgement.

Although organ transplants are an extreme example, patients meet with daily problems, such as the timing of

---

[22] http://journals.plos.org/plosone/article?id=10.1371/journal.pone.0159086

performance of an MRI scan. In a medical institution it is possible that insufficient attention is paid to the urgency or the medical circumstances requiring the specific test. It is incumbent upon the patient or his family to draw the attention of the medical team to the potential urgency, if it seems that insufficient weight was given to the circumstances of the case, instead of meekly taking a piece of paper that tells you to come back next month for the scan.

Empathy
Empathy is a critical factor in providing healthcare, and it is not a quality at which every physician excels. A 2002 study[23] concluded, among other findings, that *"Psychiatrists had the highest mean empathy score, followed by physicians in general internal medicine, general pediatrics, emergency medicine, and family medicine. The lowest means were scored by physicians in anesthesiology, orthopedic surgery, neurosurgery, radiology, and cardiovascular surgery."* Some of these results correlate well with data about unnecessary surgery (for instance, in orthopedics), which will be discussed later in this book.

When we consider that, as has been said, a lack of empathy plays a role in creating an unconscious bias (and in extreme cases when the physician really does not care about his patient at all, a conscious one), the takeaway is that we cannot blindly rely on the assessment of a surgeon that a specific surgery is not suitable for us. This may be his unconscious (or, again, conscious) way to get rid of us, dictated by his lack of empathy toward our trouble, as well as possibly by other utilitarian considerations. That fits well my experience with my father, which I related earlier in this chapter.

---

[23] "Physician empathy: definition, components, measurement, and relationship to gender and specialty" (2002). CRMEHC Faculty Papers. Paper 4. - http://jdc.jefferson.edu/crmehc/4

Takeaways from This Chapter:

► Medical bias, including ageism and gender bias, is a serious problem in the diagnosis and the treatment of patients alike.
► Medical bias will influence a patient's "informed decision" when the options presented to him are framed according to the doctor's inclinations and preferences. (See Chapter 5 for a more detailed discussion of "framing.")
► Lack of empathy in a physician is a serious problem, which may affect his judgment when deciding which therapy to recommend to a patient.

CHAPTER 3
Does That Diagnosis "Feel" Right?

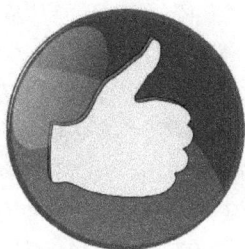

You don't have any medical training (well, maybe you do, but this book is intended for everybody, including the general public that did not go to medical school). Nevertheless, you just received a diagnosis that doesn't feel right to you. You can't pin down the reasons for your uneasiness, but it's there. **Do not discount that nagging feeling!**

Intuition is not some random thought completely disconnected from reality. A form of intuition is "skilled intuition"[24] in which a solution to a problem comes to mind quickly because familiar cues are recognized, so it is important to understand the role that our mind plays in all this.

---

[24] Gary A. Klein, *Sources of Power: How People Make Decisions*.

Have you ever thought how is it that your body is capable of running a myriad of complex biochemical reactions all the time, and to get everything running smoothly and correctly? Who is sitting in the control room of your "chemical factory" and making sure that everything is timed right? All those processes run autonomously, without the need for your intervention, because if they needed you to run them, you would die right away. Your mind doesn't need you to run the show while it processes the information needed to keep your body ticking, and does so with formidable speed. It follows that you know much more about what's going on in your body than you realize you do. Dr. Martin Rossman[25] explains that *"intuition is defined as 'power of knowing without recourse to reason' and is perceived by inner seeing, inner listening, and inner feeling. It may well be a specialized function of the right hemisphere of the brain. Through the right brain's ability to perceive subtle cues regarding feelings and connections, we are guided by what we call instincts, gut feelings, and hunches. By becoming quiet and attentive to our inner thoughts, we can use the talents of this neglected part of our minds most effectively."*

You must listen to your body because although it will never send you a detailed memo, it continuously signals to you important information about what is happening in your "chemical plant." If you choose to ignore its signals, you are missing out on what could be the most important data needed to achieve wellbeing.

A Real-life Example

I will share with you here my very personal and eye-opening experience that illustrates how intuition can sometimes keep

---

[25] Rossman, Martin L., *Guided Imagery for Self-Healing: An Essential Resource for Anyone Seeking Wellness*. New World Library. Kindle Edition.

you out of trouble. This is where I can exemplify this point with actual data that show why blindly following your doctor's prescription may be a fatal mistake. Figure 1 below is a screenshot of the readings of my albumin/creatinine ratio at the relevant testing dates (indicated beside each result—in the DD/MM/YY format).

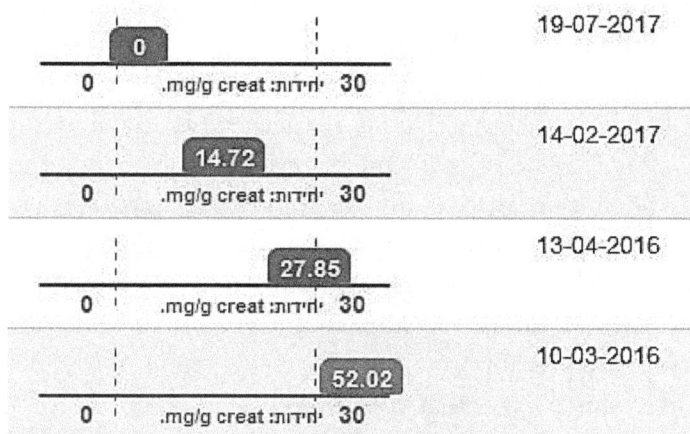

Fig. 1: Albumin/Creatinine Ratio Readings.

If you are not familiar with this ratio, what it means is that if you have a reading above 30 mg/g, you have a hidden kidney disease that, if left untreated, will destroy your kidneys. That is typical of diabetics. My reading[26] on March 10, 2016 was 52.02 mg/g, so my doctor dutifully prescribed a drug that I would take for the rest of my life. Based on what the medical literature says, her prescription was entirely reasonable and to the point. But the medical literature was not developed by studying Kfir's kidneys—it is based on statistical data of a large number of non-Kfir individuals.

---

[26] Source: Kfir's Maccabi Healthcare Online Records. Maccabi Healthcare is a leading Israeli health services provider.

I read about the drug and its side effects, and taking it didn't feel right to me. For whatever reason (let's call it intuition), I felt that I had to give my kidneys a chance before I became drug-dependent. My doctor was unhappy, but grudgingly agreed to wait one month (but no more!) and to delay treatment until the next test would convince me that I was being capricious. The next reading was high, but inside the norm, and the last reading was zero!

Had I followed my doctor's well-meaning instructions I would be taking a drug that I don't need, which has undesirable side effects, some of them quite unpleasant in the long term. This doesn't mean that my doctor's suggestions are usually wrong. On the contrary, they are usually perfectly right. I want to make it clear that I'm not suggesting that you should ignore your doctor's advice or stop taking your medicine without appropriate precautions. What I am suggesting over and over again in this book is that you should be in command of your health, question each and every conclusion and recommendation that the medical system gives you, and test your unique body's reaction, within safe and responsible limits, to achieve the best health that you can get and deserve.

I Miss My Good Old Doctor

When I saw the results that are reported in Figure 1, it immediately reminded me of Dr. Horowitz, a doctor I had once (too many years ago to mention). He was an old-school family physician, who had learned his trade in South Africa and had possibly the best bedside manners I have ever seen. One day I got the results of a comprehensive blood test that he had talked me into doing after long negotiations, and one result was very bad, high above the norm. I ran to my doctor with the piece of paper, feeling (obviously unreasonably) that it was all his fault for having convinced me to do this screening in the first place. He was, as usual, unruffled.

"All other results are fine. This probably doesn't mean anything. Do another test next week," he said.

"And what if the result is still bad then?" I asked accusingly.

"Repeat until normal!" he said.

I didn't appreciate at the time how much sense this advice makes in some cases. The trick, of course, is to know when it doesn't make sense. We will be talking about RUN (repeat until normal) again, later in this book.

Why Intuition Matters

Patient intuition is not nonsense and it has both beneficial and deleterious potential, which means that it should not be ignored by the treating physician (which unfortunately is often the case). Physicians may not like it and brush it aside as meaningless, which in many cases it may be. But on the other hand, in some cases it may play a critical role. This very question was reviewed in a paper by Buetow and Mintoft,[27] which summarizes the point by explaining that *"Illness beliefs, including intuitions, and the trajectory of the illness experience interact through psychophysiological relationships. Nerve cells receive sensory inputs that may undergo automatic preconscious evaluation. A general sense of the stimulus is fed back to perceptual centers, which generate a response that can have a bodily expression."*

In other words, we may not know what is actually going on inside, but we may feel "something," some kind of uneasiness that tells us that, somewhere, something bad is going on. Should we or our doctor ignore it? Certainly not. As the review further

---

[27] When Should Patient Intuition be Taken Seriously? Stephen A. Buetow, PhD and Bridget Mintoft, MSocSc (Hons), Dip Psych (Clin) - https://www.ncbi.nlm.nih.gov/pmc/articles/PMC3055972

explains, *"... patients ... can, for example, produce complex schemas that reflect their awareness of patterned change in their bodies or the bodies of others, as when a mother strongly senses her child is unwell. ... The accuracy of these types of intuition may increase with patients' explicit (conscious) learning; their implicit (unconscious) learning through focused attention on their environment; the duration and repetition of their experience; and feedback from the environment. Sharing intuitive knowledge with the clinician can help the clinician make a differential diagnosis and manage concerns."*

But there is another reason, beyond aiding in the diagnosis of a condition, that makes it imperative for a clinician to listen to his patient: Intuition of one's medical condition may influence the patient's perception of the illness, which in turn may have a negative (or positive) effect on the outcome. This subject was reviewed in a paper by Petrie and coworkers,[28] in which the authors relate that *"... the number of symptoms the patient associates with their condition or illness identity was predictive of future healthcare use in the following 6 months. These studies highlight the importance of the patient's beliefs and emotional responses to their symptoms and illness as key factors influencing satisfaction with the consultation and the future use of health care."*

So what happens when you share intuitive thoughts about your condition with your doctor, and he pushes them aside? If your intuitions do not align well with the doctor's diagnosis and they have not been seriously considered and explained away, you will continue to worry and to live with a perception of your condition that is not the same as the diagnosis, either as regards the severity or the nature of your condition. Regardless of the fact that your intuition and the resulting illness perception may

---

[28] https://www.fmhs.auckland.ac.nz/assets/fmhs/som/psychmed/petrie/docs/2007_IPsPetrieCurrOpinPsy.pdf

be 100% wrong, and your doctor may be 100% right, research shows that this situation will adversely affect the outcome of your treatment, creating a nocebo effect,[29] defined as "a harmless substance or treatment that when taken by or administered to a patient is associated with harmful side effects or worsening of symptoms due to negative expectations or the psychological condition of the patient."

As Jo Marchant points out,[30] *"Warning patients about pain or discomfort they are about to feel is a staple of conventional medical care. But Lang argues that during medical procedures such as scans or operations, we are particularly susceptible to the nocebo effect, and that being told how much things are about to hurt simply worsens our pain."* But being left to stew with our own doubts and worries is the self-serving equivalent of that situation.

Lissa Rankin[31] takes this a step further, arguing that in many cases you can rely on your intuition as a tool to heal yourself. As she puts it, *"Your Inner Pilot Light, the wise healer that lies within you, is your body's best friend and always knows exactly what your body needs. But many have unwittingly distanced themselves from the wisdom of their Inner Pilot Lights. Often, this is because we no longer reside in our own bodies. Instead of living embodied lives, heeding the wisdom of our intuition, and feeling all five senses in our own skin, we dissociate."* While I certainly agree that listening to your body is important and that understanding certain problems may be the key to solving them (we will discuss this more with reference to psychosomatic conditions), I am certainly not suggesting that it

---

[29] For a detailed discussion of the nocebo effect, see Chapter 10.

[30] Marchant, Jo. *Cure: A Journey into the Science of Mind Over Body* (pp. 124–125).

[31] Rankin M.D., Lissa. *Mind Over Medicine: Scientific Proof That You Can Heal Yourself.*

is possible to attempt to cure every condition, or even the majority of them, using hypnosis or guided imagery. Those are extremely important and very effective tools in many cases, (both as the major solution of psychosomatic conditions and a supporting factor in conventional therapy, as well as in the prevention of stress-related conditions), but are not even close to being a universal solution.

The Lost Power to Make Decisions

Our ability to make sensible assessments and to reach reasonable conclusions regarding our health has been taken away from us because the message we receive from the system is that it is no longer needed, that it is an old skill no longer useful in modern days. We need to reclaim it. The instinctive reaction of every parent to waking up at night with a little child who is barking while coughing, is to put on some clothes and run with him to the nearest ER, where he will most likely be told that this is stridor caused by croup (a result of common cold) and if it hasn't already passed by the time they get to the ER, it will disappear shortly. We could have taken the child out, to breathe some cool air, and gone back to bed in a few minutes instead of hanging around hospitals (that's what experienced parents do).

But it wasn't always like that, because in the past parents didn't have ERs to run to at the slightest provocation. Flash back to the beginning of last century; much of the world's population didn't have quick and easy access to medical care. Many lived in rural areas, far away from the nearest doctor, and had to make decisions and sometimes fateful ones. To them, the 1833 booklet by Mrs. Child, titled *The American Frugal Housewife*,[32] came in handy, because of its chapter on "Simple

---

[32] *The American Frugal Housewife*, by Mrs. Child, Twelfth Edition, Carter, Boston - Hendee, and Co., 1833 – See Appendix 2.

Remedies." It teaches us, for instance, to cure dysentery—a condition that nowadays would have us running to the ER—by drinking a spoonful of a mixture of table-salt in keen vinegar in a gill[33] of boiling water. I can't testify as to the efficacy of this remedy, but the point is that people were expected, when called upon to deal with an emergency, to take matters in their own hands.

The more "modern" 1900 reference book, *The Cottage Physician*,[34] instructs us on many things, among them, how to administer a "proper treatment" to someone who has become paralyzed. Of course, nobody in his right mind would nowadays attempt to treat a case of paralysis at home, but the point is that we have gone to the opposite extreme by stopping to think on our own and by delegating all the decisions to a medical system that may often be great, but in some cases is disastrous. We have been taught that we cannot and should not interfere with medical decisions and should simply do as we are told. I believe that, as is true in many cases, the middle course is the right one, as discussed throughout this book.

In order to bring us back to the reality of life, since it may happen that no immediate medical assistance is available (say, for instance, if you are all alone in the middle of a desert), it is worth referring for the last time to Mrs. Child's advice:

> *As this book may fall into the hands of those who cannot speedily obtain a physician, it is worth while to mention what is best to be done for the bite of a rattlesnake:—Cut the flesh out, around the bite, **instantly**; that the poison may not have the time to circulate in the blood. If caustic is at hand, put it upon the raw flesh; if not, the next best*

---

[33] A gill is a quarter of a pint.
[34] *The Cottage Physician*, The King-Richardson Co., Springfield, Mass, 1900 – See Appendix 3.

thing is to fill the wound with salt—renewing it occasionally. Take a dose of sweet oil and spirits of turpentine, to defend the stomach. If the whole limb swell, bathe it in salt and vinegar freely. It is well to physic the system thoroughly, before returning to usual diet.

It is indeed sobering to think of how things happened in 1833, and how we have been pampered by modern medicine. However, our destiny is still in our hands, in spite of the fact that the medical system gives us the tools, the support, and the knowledge that was not available back then. I do not expect that readers of this book will have much call for handling a rattlesnake bite, but this will remind us that, in many different ways, we are still on our own.

Takeaways from This Chapter:

▶ You must always listen to your body. The signals it sends you may be difficult to decipher and the reasons for your uneasiness may not be easily understood, but if one is there, it should be heeded.

▶ The medical system has become so complex and specialized that we inevitably feel that we have lost our power to make important decisions about our health. That is a role that we must reclaim.

▶ Participating in our health decisions does not mean ignoring what our doctor tells us, but it means not allowing your doctor to ignore our questions, intuitions, and suggestions.

CHAPTER 4
Is Mine a Widespread Condition?

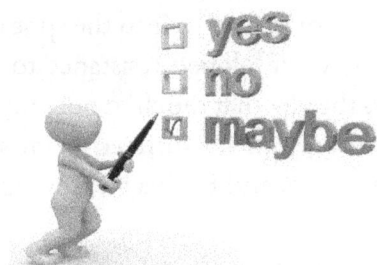

Many common conditions are misdiagnosed on a daily basis, for a variety of reasons. Many mistakes can be attributed to the effect that Professor Kahneman calls "What You See Is All There Is" (WYSIATI).[35] This effect is what makes you or your doctor jump to conclusions on the basis of limited evidence. Because sometimes your symptoms are similar to those of a "fashionable" condition, your doctor may be tempted to jump to a diagnosis that fits the evidence he has, in spite of the fact that additional evidence would have changed that diagnosis. Even worse—we may be influenced by the fact that we know of

---

[35] Kahneman, Daniel. *Thinking, Fast and Slow* (p. 85).

other people who have been diagnosed with a widespread condition, into believing that our own symptoms mean that we have it too. In such a situation we may subconsciously suppress tale-telling symptoms of an altogether different condition, and mislead our doctor by glorifying others. Whether our doctor will see through it is the difference between a good and a bad physician. But if we are aware that this might be the case, we may help him get to the bottom of our actual illness.

Anybody who has raised children in the past 30 years or so knows how easily pediatricians used to prescribe antibiotics to kids who had a viral infection (to which antibiotics do nothing whatsoever), on the strength of a red throat or ear, and one temperature reading. The overuse of antibiotics made under the WYSIATI effect famously got us into the spot we are in today, where pathogens have developed resistance to many of them. And that's besides the fact that the child not only did not benefit from taking the drug, but he suffered from side effects, for instance, to his stomach, and from a weakening of his immune system.

Thus, if on the basis of limited information you are told that your symptoms are likely to be those of common indigestion, please make sure that you are not having a heart attack instead. And speaking of heart attacks, if you really need to get one, you'd better be a male, and old, because young people are less likely to have chest pain; also, heart attacks are much more misdiagnosed in females than in men. A recent study[36] showed that *"Among younger adults with acute coronary syndrome, women and men had different access to care. Moreover, fewer than half of men and women with ST-segment elevation MI received timely primary coronary intervention. Our results also highlight that men and women with no chest pain and*

_____

[36] http://www.cmaj.ca/content/cmaj/early/2014/03/17/cmaj. 131450.full.pdf

those with anxiety, several traditional risk factors and feminine personality traits were at particularly increased risk of poorer access to care."

On the other hand, you may be diagnosed with a heart attack when, in fact, your problem is altogether different. In Chapter 1 I already mentioned pulmonary embolism, which is caused by a blood clot. Pulmonary embolism is a blockage of the pulmonary artery, the main artery in the lung. Symptoms include sharp chest pain, shortness of breath, fainting, and anxiety. A 2013 study found that 55% of patients with pulmonary embolism were sent home or admitted to hospitals with a wrong diagnosis, causing many cases of death. Pulmonary embolism can be mistaken for other conditions such as a heart attack or pneumonia.

It is not that clogged coronary arteries are a rarity. Mortality from ischemic heart disease is the single largest cause of death worldwide, which in 2008 caused 7,249,000 deaths,[37] or 12.7% of total global mortality. And still, amazingly, it gets misdiagnosed. Thus, as discussed in the previous chapter, if the ER doctor tells you that it looks like you are having an anxiety attack, or may have eaten something that disagreed with you, take a good look at that intuition that brought you to the ER in the first place, and insist on getting more meaningful tests than a doctor's cursory examination.

Misdiagnosing a Drug Side Effect for a Disease

It so happens that ER doctors are seldom luminaries. I have learned that very clearly when I was rushed to the ER because, out of the blue, I had started spurting blood from my nose. My blood pressure was at a whopping 260/130mmHg and I was

---

[37] https://www.ncbi.nlm.nih.gov/pmc/articles/PMC3819990/pdf/main.pdf

immediately given medication to lower it. I was flattered to see that two doctors, a middle-aged man and a younger woman, were taking an interest in my case. After a while they came to my bed and handed me a piece of paper.

"What is this?" I asked.

"This is a prescription for the medicines that you need to take from now on."

I looked at the list, in which I recognized a beta-blocker and a diuretic. A couple of other drugs were new to me, but I was acutely aware of the unpleasant side effects of beta blockers.[38] I gave the doctors an inquisitive look.

"Listen," said the older one, "I know that this is a shock to you, but your blood pressure is dangerously high and you must make peace with it and take your medication, or else ..."

I have been a 110/70 person all my life, so that extreme jump in my blood pressure didn't make sense to me. I searched my head for a clue, and then the penny dropped.

"I think I know what's going on," I said. "I have been taking an NSAID drug for my lower back pain for a week now. I remember skimming through the patient information in the accompanying leaflet, and reading that it may cause high blood pressure. That must be it," I suggested.

(The patient leaflet actually says: "This medicine may lead to an increase in blood pressure, and so your doctor may ask to monitor your blood pressure on a regular basis.")

Both doctors gave me a compassionate look, as if to say that I was clutching at straws.

---

[38] Dizziness, weakness, drowsiness or fatigue, cold hands and feet, dry mouth, skin, or eyes, headache, upset stomach, diarrhea or constipation, depression, shortness of breath, wheezing or trouble breathing, loss of sex drive/erectile dysfunction (ED), trouble sleeping, swelling of the hands or feet, slow heartbeat, skin rash, sore throat, memory loss or confusion, back or joint pain.

"I never heard of this," said the older one.

"No, that's not it," said the other, speaking decisively and authoritatively. "Please make sure to take your medication daily and in a week talk to your doctor for a refill."

That, of course, made my confidence in my explanation waver. I thanked them, took my prescription and went home, where I re-read the patient leaflet and found that my memory had served me well. I stopped taking the NSAID and three days later my blood pressure was back to normal. I threw away the prescription that I had kept to be on the safe side.

Isn't the modern medical system wonderful?

Celiac Disease

According to Rachel Begun, MS, RDN,[39] it is estimated that 83% of Americans who have celiac disease (CD) are undiagnosed or misdiagnosed with other conditions. On the other hand, a (limited) 2009 study[40] found an opposite result, i.e., *"... a high rate of histological and serological misdiagnosis of CD ... mainly due to a histological overdiagnosis of CD."* This result was confirmed by a broader 2016 study, which concluded that *"... our study shows that a considerable number of patients referred to a tertiary care center experience previous misdiagnosis and/or overdiagnosis of CD."*

The net result is that in many cases the diagnosis of CD, or failure to diagnose it, may be a severe hazard for the patient, because as time passes a celiac patient who continues to eat gluten may worsen his or her situation. This is more complex, because gluten is bad for you, whether you have CD or not. As

---

[39] https://www.beyondceliac.org/celiac-disease/facts-and-figures
[40] https://www.researchgate.net/publication/41547332
_Very_high_rate_of_misdiagnosis_of_celiac_disease_in_clinical_practice

Dr. Davis points out in his book,[41] gluten does not come alone but is mainly derived from wheat, and *"A complex range of diseases results from consumption of wheat, from celiac disease—the devastating intestinal disease that develops from exposure to wheat gluten—to an assortment of neurological disorders, diabetes, heart disease, arthritis, curious rashes, and the paralyzing delusions of schizophrenia."*

CD is also most often misdiagnosed as irritable bowel syndrome (IBS). IBS is associated with an overly sensitive colon, or large intestine. People with IBS seem to have trouble with the movement in their colon. In some cases, contents in the colon move too fast and the colon doesn't absorb enough fluid, which causes diarrhea. In other cases, the contents don't move fast enough and too much fluid is absorbed, causing constipation. This is unpleasant, but it is not CD, and if someone with IBS is misdiagnosed with CD, he is not getting the right treatment. Since a pillar of CD treatment is the avoidance of gluten, a person suffering from IBS may find himself eating foods containing gluten substitutes, which are bad stuff. As Dr. Davis explains, many gluten-free foods are made by replacing wheat flour with cornstarch, rice starch, potato starch, or tapioca starch (starch extracted from the root of the cassava plant). This is especially hazardous for anybody looking to drop some weight, since gluten-free foods, though they do not trigger the immune or neurological response of wheat gluten, still trigger the glucose-insulin response that causes you to gain weight. Wheat products increase blood sugar and insulin more than most other foods, but foods made with cornstarch, rice starch, potato starch, and tapioca starch are among the few foods that increase blood sugar even more than wheat products. Thus, in

---

[41] Davis MD, William. *Wheat Belly: Lose the Wheat, Lose the Weight, and Find Your Path Back to Health.*

seeking to avoid one problem that you may not have, you may be running into an altogether different one.

Many More Misdiagnosed Diseases

The intention of this chapter is not to provide an exhaustive list of commonly misdiagnosed diseases. There are many others: For instance, a 2014 article published by the John Hopkins School of Medicine[42] maintains that doctors overlook or discount early signs of potentially disabling strokes in tens of thousands of Americans each year. A large number of missed strokes occurs in visitors to ERs who complain of dizziness or headaches but are sent home. Women, minorities, and people under the age of 45 are significantly more likely to be misdiagnosed. There are many other examples ranging from easily treatable problems like thyroid imbalance, to more serious ones such as cancer. The variety is great, including autoimmune conditions, such as multiple sclerosis, rheumatoid arthritis, and lupus, which may be misdiagnosed as depression or viral illness, and Lyme disease, which may be misdiagnosed as mononucleosis, flu, and depression, or migraine, which may be misdiagnosed as a brain tumor, aneurysm, and stroke.

This chapter is only meant to give you an idea of what may happen and has hopefully convinced you not to submit passively to whatever diagnosis is presented to you. Remember: Your life may depend on your willingness to probe and on your strength, if needed, to contest that diagnosis. If you truly feel that something is wrong with the diagnosis and discuss this openly (and relentlessly) with your doctor, there is a good chance that he will invest more time and thought in it. Nobody wants to be found at fault for mistreating a patient who has told

---

[42] https://www.hopkinsmedicine.org/news/media/releases/ er_doctors_commonly_miss_more_strokes_among_women_minorities_a nd_younger_patients

him so. And if your doctor will hate you for being insistent ... well, that's his tough luck.

Takeaways from This Chapter:

▶ Knowing that an illness is currently widespread may create a bias in both the physician's and the patient's minds, leading to a wrong diagnosis.
▶ Many diseases are misdiagnosed, at times with dire consequences. To increase our chances of avoiding a wrong diagnosis we must be inquisitive and, if needed, ready to contest a diagnosis that we believe wrong, no matter why.

CHAPTER 5
How Will Treatment Impact My Life?

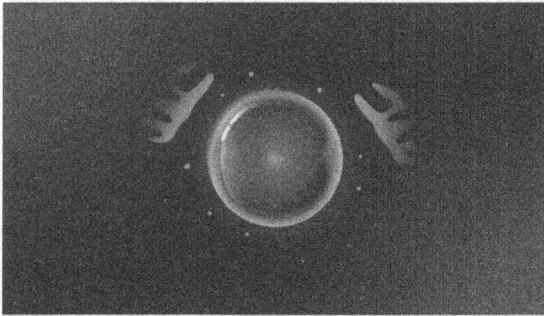

Decisions that we make regarding a medical treatment that we are about to receive impact not only the resolution of our medical problem, but often also the quality of our life thereafter. That's another reason why making the right decision is so critical, but unfortunately we are likely to make wrong decisions most of the time, because of the faulty decision-making process discussed by Kahneman.[43] This happens when we are asked to decide between different options such as alternative therapies (including not doing anything and going

---

[43] See Chapter 1.

on as we are), without having the specific knowledge needed to do so. We may make an impulsive decision that in retrospective was clearly wrong but at the time seemed to be the right thing to do. Let's examine in some detail how this happens.

First, our decision can be influenced by the doctor who is presenting our choices to us and by his personal preferences that result in a particular presentation, in what is known as a "framing effect." The following example will illustrate the point. Assume that you have a condition that is not life-threatening, but it bothers you daily and makes your life miserable—for instance, a recurring crippling pain in your lower back. A specialist—Doctor A—gives you these options:

You can choose a surgical procedure that in 98% of the cases rids the patient of the problem altogether and only has a very low incidence of side effects; or

You can choose to take a drug for the rest of your life, bearing in mind that 60% of the patients find that medication does not solve the problem or only relieves it partially.

Chances are that you will choose to undergo surgery, because of the very high success rate and because you feel that taking drugs every day of your life, when the failure rate of this treatment is so high, would not be a smart choice. Makes sense so far.

If, instead, you are seeing Doctor B, however, your options may be explained to you in this way:

You can choose a surgical procedure that although it has a high success rate, in 2% of the cases leaves the patient in a wheelchair with irreparable nervous damage; or

You can choose to take medication with only light side effects, if any. Forty percent of the patients are quite happy with the results and in much larger numbers at least some meaningful improvement is felt. Of course, if it should become necessary, it is always possible to stop medication and try surgery.

If your physician is Doctor B, you are very likely to choose drug therapy, because the danger of finding yourself in a wheelchair is so frightening that a 2% chance seems substantial. On the other hand, if the drug doesn't work you still have your options open, so it makes sense to try that route first.

But if you check the example carefully, you will see that both presentations reflect the exact same situation and yet, in spite of that, they have brought you to diametrically opposite decisions. What you are seeing is the effect of framing. Doctor A is a surgeon, so he has framed it from the point of view of someone who is sympathetic to surgery, while Doctor B is a general practitioner who cures people with medicines every day.

You may be asking yourself which decision is more likely to be wrong, and the answer would be that either one, or perhaps both are wrong, because you are asked to make a decision without being provided with sufficient data, so you are using your intuition to decide. When you use your intuition in things of such importance, you are likely to end up wrong. Your doctor, however, will feel good because he has explained the options to you and has given you the data "you need" to make a decision. After all, it is the patient's right to be told everything the physician thinks is relevant and to make the final decision.

According to the American Medical Association Code of Medical Ethics,[44] *"Informed consent to medical treatment is fundamental in both ethics and law. Patients have the right to receive information and ask questions about recommended treatments so that they can make well-considered decisions about care."* The principle is right and admirable, but it is often difficult to put into practice because although the physician is required to *"present relevant information accurately and sensitively, in keeping with the patient's preferences for receiving medical information,"* he has no way to be sure how well the patient appreciates *the meaning* of the information given him, particularly if repression is involved. Even though what the physician must give him includes *"the diagnosis (when known), the nature and purpose of recommended interventions, and the burdens, risks, and expected benefits of all options, including forgoing treatment,"* unless the patient has a medical background, or has educated himself on the subject (see Chapter 11 – Your Survival Kit), a substantial component of his decision-making process will still be intuition.

When you are called upon to make a decision in a situation in which you don't have sufficient information, the outcome is influenced by utterly irrelevant factors. In this example, those irrelevant factors could be, for instance, the authoritative tone of voice of the physician, the doctor's reputation that you have heard whispered by a friend of a friend of yours, or even his or her looks. Lacking solid data, you will unconsciously look for factors that will justify your intuitive (and, very likely, wrong) decision. However, whether your outcome will be a positive one or not, is left entirely to luck.

---

[44] https://www.ama-assn.org/delivering-care/informed-consent

Here is a not dissimilar example. Assume that you wake up in a strange hotel. You arrived late at night and didn't have the time, the interest, or the strength to tour the hotel and get acquainted with its topography. However, it was the fire alarm that woke you up and your room is now in flames. You have to get out, but to do so you must choose between two doors, one of which leads to safety and the other will get you trapped in the burning hotel. How do you choose between the doors? You look for hints in them that may tell you which one leads out. The two doors look different but equally uninformatively so. You look at the doorknobs and at the markings on the floor for hints that will tell you which one is used more frequently. One may also look slightly more ornate than the other. The frequency of use is totally irrelevant to the problem with which you are confronted, and so is the ornamental level of the door, but you must make a decision and you need to rationalize to yourself why you are choosing one door over the other, while you have no other information available to you. The outcome is left to luck.

Now to look at it from another angle, let's slightly rephrase the description given by Doctor A:

You can choose a surgical procedure that rids 98 out of 100 patients of the problem altogether and only has a very low incidence of side effects; or

You can choose to take a drug for the rest of your life, bearing in mind that 60 out of 100 patients find that medication does not solve the problem or only relieves it partially.

Now making a decision to take the surgery has become more difficult, hasn't it? The reason is that now you don't see an impersonal statistic (a percentage), you see **people**. When you hear that 98 out of 100 patients have a successful surgery you cannot help thinking of the poor two patients who failed. After all, two patients are much more real than 2% of the patients, and you could be one of those two. You wonder whether enduring all the pain would be worth it. You can visualize yourself suffering after the unsuccessful surgery and you can feel the pain. That thought naturally bothers you and makes you think much more about the whole matter. That's why doctors speak in percentages—the statistic dehumanizes the issue and makes the conversation much simpler and more sterile. No physician wants an excited and hard-thinking patient on his hands. That's also why you must be very careful when information is presented to you in terms of percentages. I always joke with doctors when talking about medical statistics, that a 50% success of a procedure means that one patient died and the other one is yet to die. It is a (noir) joke indeed, but sometimes it is not so far from reality. Statistics can be manipulated and are often used by people who don't understand them properly. That's why it is not uncommon to read review papers that criticize articles they have reviewed, pointing out that their conclusions are a result of the poor statistical significance of their data.

What Happens after Therapy
Now assume that after listening to either Doctor A or Doctor B you go home and do your homework. You find that a set of physical exercises done daily is said to substantially reduce lower back pain. From the blogs you read, people seem to describe a pain quite similar to your own. Now which therapy will you be inclined to take, that preferred by Doctor A or by Doctor B?

Some people will tell both doctors "no thank you" and try their hand at physical therapy first. That, however, is the easy answer to the question and we can't always come up with easy answers, so let's take a different look at the matter. What does the fact that 98% of the patients no longer suffer from lower back pains tell you about the quality of your life after surgery? Nothing, of course. Assume for a moment (a not completely imaginary scenario) that the surgery requires inserting rods in your back that will stiffen it. You will no longer be able to bend forward as you did before, and your range of motion will be severely limited. Yes, your lower back will no longer ache (if you are lucky), but how appealing is that surgery now?

There is no doubt that your doctor will make a full disclosure to you regarding all the potential negative results, and it is almost certain that you will discount them as something that "happens to other people." After all, your doctor is so competent and full of confidence, and the future that awaits you after a successful surgery looks so rosy ...

But you must be aware of the long-term implications of surgery. Take for instance bariatric surgery,[45] which is a commonly employed solution to severe obesity. It may save the patient from the terrible implications of obesity, but it may also cause some baffling long-term complications, such as neuropathies due to nutritional deficiencies, internal hernias, anastomotic stenoses, and emotional disorders. Patients may also encounter side effects such as difficulties in swallowing, which are not life-threatening but have meaningful quality-of-life issues. Unless you have read extensively on the subject before agreeing to undergo surgery, gathering information from different sources looking at the subject from different angles,

---

[45] https://www.ncbi.nlm.nih.gov/pmc/articles/PMC2729256/

you are unlikely to have a full appreciation of the meaning of all that on your life from now on.

Reasons Why Doctors Love a Therapy

There are many reasons why a doctor loves one therapy more than another and therefore tends to offer it preferentially. Some such reasons (ordered from the best to the worse) are:

- He believes it is the best option for you.
- He has had a high rate of success with it in the past, and he sees is no reason to change winning horses.
- His clinic/hospital/ward is equipped to administer that therapy and not so much for the alternative one.
- He has not kept himself sufficiently informed about the alternative option.
- He has received a grant to do research using that particular therapy.
- If he can talk you into doing that particular therapy privately, he will make more money from it.

There can obviously be other reasons, such as he may simply be a bad doctor, incompetent, and/or indolent, but let's see how we deal with this reality. It is not enough that the treating physician comes recommended by your doctor, your friends, or a blog on the Internet. Strange as it may seem at first sight, you need to assess your doctor to get a feel for his level of interest in your problem, his span of attention, and his openness toward your questions. You must see if he is too confident or too insecure, if his is a one-track mind or he is considering different options. Although at times, when you are particularly vulnerable, you may look upon your doctor as a savior, you must remember that he is not God—he is a service supplier, and as such he must give you the confidence that he is the right one for you. Just like you would not pick a nanny for your child if she didn't inspire confidence, you shouldn't follow a physician's opinion unless you have "interviewed" him and are satisfied with the answers you got. Chapter 11 includes suggestions on how to inquire, with information at hand.

Takeaways from This Chapter:

▶ Regardless of whether your direct problem has been fixed by a treatment, your life may never be the same. It doesn't pay to fix a nagging pain in your knee, for example, if as a result of surgery complications you now have a respiratory problem.

▶ When mulling your options, never look at the chances of success in terms of percentages. Always translate those percentages into real numbers and think what they mean for you if you end up on the wrong side of the equation.

▶ Keep in mind that physicians coming from different disciplines are likely to frame your problem and therapy in different ways, which may lead to diametrically opposite conclusions.

CHAPTER 6
Case Study: Type 2 Diabetes

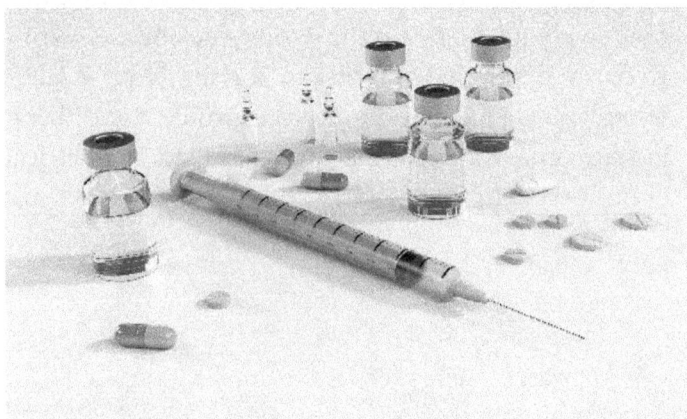

There are several reasons why I have taken type 2 diabetes as a case study here:

◆ Type 2 diabetes is a very common and widespread condition that is widely mistreated;

◆ I have personal experience with its mistreatment, but have eventually reversed my condition; and

◆ it tells you a lot about the pitfalls of the medical system.

It all started when I woke up one morning with an astronomic HbA1C (glycated hemoglobin[46]) of 12.1 and a fasting glucose level of 312 mg/dl. With those numbers, I had to do something immediately, or I was in line for hideous diseases and premature death. My doctor immediately placed me on strong medication. As a result, only three months later, on June 21, 2016, my fasting blood sugar level had dropped to 138 mg/dl and my HbA1C to a mere 6%. That's great, right? **Wrong!**

Fast forward eight months to February 14, 2017. My fasting blood sugar level had gone up to 157 mg/dl, and my HbA1C to 6.8%. The efficacy of the treatment was obviously diminishing, and I started to recall people telling me that, once you start on the path of blood sugar medication, you may end up injecting insulin. I wasn't going to take that lying down.

When you become diabetic, you want to think that it is an act of God, that you are not responsible for it. It's just the world being mean to you. But while obviously in some cases diabetes may be due to your genetic makeup or to other causes over which you have no control, that's untrue for most people. The reading and reasoning that I had done over the months since that fateful morning in March had convinced me that I had been causing it to myself with my own actions. I had been overeating and, what's worse, eating the wrong kinds of food. I was overweight and wasn't exercising enough. I reasoned that what I did to myself I might perhaps undo, if I could just find and follow the right path.

It took me five more months to prove that I was right and that managing my blood sugar level without taking drugs was possible. After stopping taking medication altogether for three and a half months (after a thorough, responsible, and careful

---

[46] HbA1C, also referred to simply as "A1C," is a form of hemoglobin that is measured primarily to identify the three-month average plasma glucose concentration.

priming period), I took a new blood test, on July 19, 2017. My fasting blood sugar was 102 mg/dl and my HbA1C was 5.8%.

My fasting glucose levels (Fig. 2) and HbA1C levels (Fig. 3) are shown below. For reference, note that I stopped taking glucose-lowering medication on April 4, 2017 (dates in the tables are in the DD/MM/YY format):

102 mg/dl	19-07-2017
157 mg/dl	14-02-2017
138 mg/dl	07-08-2016
312 mg/dl	10-03-2016

Fig. 2: Fasting Glucose Levels.
Source: Kfir's Maccabi Healthcare Online Records

5.8 % Total Hb.	19-07-2017
6.8 % Total Hb.	14-02-2017
6 % Total Hb.	21-06-2016
12.1 % Total Hb.	10-03-2016

Fig. 3: HbA1C Levels.
Source: Kfir's Maccabi Healthcare Online Records

Since then, my HbA1C level has gone down further to 5.7 and I expect it to continue to improve with time. A detailed explanation of how I accomplished this result exceeds the scope of this book and is related elsewhere.[47] For now, suffice it to understand that it can be done, but that's not the direction in which the medical system pointed me.

---

[47] Luzzatto, Kfir; *How to Reverse Your Diabetes (If You Really Mean It)*.

At the outset, when my blood sugar went skyrocketing, my doctor immediately prescribed blue pills, which she tooted as the best and most modern solution to my type 2 diabetes. She didn't sit with me and suggest that I should try first to lower my blood sugar through exercise and a diet. She didn't say, "Try this and try that and then come to me to report on the progress that you are making." She didn't ask me if I was stressed, what I was eating, and, in general, what was going on with me. She didn't think about it, not because she is a bad doctor—in fact, she is a great doctor in comparison to many others that I have known. However, she was never trained to do what it takes to guide me through my plight. She is conditioned to work exactly as the system requires of her and she doesn't have the time, knowledge, or freedom to work outside the very specific guidelines that someone who doesn't know me from Adam has drafted for a case like mine.

You could ask yourself what you would prefer: becoming drug-dependent, or going to the gym. Even if you are not excited about exercising, I believe that you would take the gym over the pill any time. So did I.

The Placebo Effect

I touched lightly on the nocebo effect before. The placebo effect is the opposite and is something that is starting to be better utilized in recent years. As Jo Marchand relates in her excellent book,[48] *"placebo effects have only been studied in a few systems so far, but there are probably many others…the placebo effect isn't a single phenomenon but a 'melting pot' of responses, each using different ingredients from the brain's natural pharmacy."* In other words, when we give a patient a placebo it is a cue for the brain to release materials that do the job, even though we were only given a sugar

---

[48] Marchant, Jo. *Cure: A Journey into the Science of Mind Over Body* (p. 17). Crown/Archetype.

pill. But the most surprising effect of all is the fact that placebo pills have a curative effect even when we know beforehand that they contain no drug! One of the leaders in this field of research is Harvard medical professor Ted Kaptchuk, who explained his results in a recent interview[49] that is worth reading. I mention this topic here simply because a good and judicious use of the placebo effect can be of help in overcoming medical conditions that can be treated without drugs, such as type 2 diabetes.

This shouldn't surprise us because healing rituals have been around since the dawn of time. As was said before, our brain runs the show and can tell our body's chemical factory to make chemical "products" that have a curative effect, but before it does so it must know that this is needed. A ritual—including that of taking a pill that admittedly contains no active material—appears to be a way to communicate that need to our brain. That's why I find that taking some food supplements in the first, psychologically intense stages of our fight with type 2 diabetes, may have a value.

Why Diabetes Drugs Are Harmful

Before we are able to appreciate how misguided the procedure adopted by the medical profession is, according to which anyone with type 2 diabetes must immediately be put on medication instead of painstakingly exploring first whether he can overcome the illness without them, we need to go into some details, so please bear with me.

Let me tell you a short fictional story in which you feature as the hero or heroine.

Your home is located at the edge of a beautiful wood. Unfortunately, the wood is inhabited by wolves, and because you inadvertently forgot to close the backdoor leading from the

[49] https://www.vox.com/science-and-health/2017/6/1/15711814/open-label-placebo-kaptchuk

outside into your basement, a pack of them has selected it for their lair. Since no barrier exists between the basement and your living room, the presence of the wolves naturally has raised concerns.

You consulted with a wolf expert, who gave you two options: the first involved going down into the basement and chasing the wolves away. You didn't find that option appealing. But luckily, the expert offered you an alternative option: to keep the wolves happy in the basement by feeding them meat tidbits on a daily basis, so they won't feel the urge to come up to your living room.

As time passed, more wolves found their way to the basement and the daily ration of meat had to be increased to keep the growing population of wolves happy and unwilling to leave the basement. And as time passed, the amount of meat you fed them became larger and larger, until one day ...

Well, one day the basement became so crowded that the meat you served the wolves no longer sufficed to keep them happy in that cramped space. They had to come up for air. They invaded your living quarters, tearing everything, you included, to pieces.

Apologies for the gritty description, but it fits quite well with what happens to your body when you decide to start taking diabetes medication. The wolves represent the glucose in your body, the meat is insulin, and the basement represents your body's cells. Let's take a closer look at that, and while we do it, let's also kill some sacred cows.

Your measurable blood sugar level is not the problem. It is a symptom of the problem. The problem is the excess glucose stored in your body but not in your bloodstream.

Hiding the symptom does not solve the problem. The fact that you managed to keep the wolves in the basement didn't make them go away, pretty much like keeping the glucose in your bloodstream low doesn't make the glucose in your body cells go away.

Diabetes medications exacerbate the problem. This is something that doctors don't tell you. Diabetes medications don't cure the illness and don't keep it static—they make it worse! They help your body to store more glucose in its cells, and thus help you to hide the problem from yourself and from your blood tests, but all the while your body is piling up sugar (by the action of the insulin—more about that later), just like dropping more meat down the basement only helps the population of wolves to grow.

Sticking your head in the sand will eventually blow up in your face. You will reach a point where your insulin resistance is so severe that your pills will no longer manage to mask your illness. Glucose will spill into your bloodstream, and your medication will no longer be able to stuff it into your already overstuffed cells. That amounts to letting the wolves out.

Shocking, isn't it? But unless you are told the hard, frightening truth, you will never resolve to do what it takes to reverse your diabetes: to clean your body of excess glucose, to stop stuffing it in the meanders of your body and hiding it from your blood tests, to improve insulin efficacy by reducing insulin resistance, and to live a reasonable life that takes all that into account.

All the bad things that diabetes drugs do

I'll say it again, because to some people this is counterintuitive: **Diabetes drugs don't cure diabetes**. They don't keep the disease static. They make it worse. They hide the symptoms and allow you to ignore your disease so it gets worse. They keep your doctor happy because he can say to himself that he has done a good job, and the alleged proof is your blood test. So the drugs keep you in a fool's paradise.

The symptom of that problem—a high level of glucose in your bloodstream—is in itself the ultimate cause of many diseases that damage your inner organs. Glucose will find its way to all parts of your body, creating a host of hideous diseases. I don't need to go into those; you know them well enough, and that's why you were quick to accept that you needed blood glucose-lowering (i.e., diabetes) treatment. But the glucose in your bloodstream is not the original problem, just like the wolf who will attack you is not the original problem. The original problem is that you let the wolf into your basement. If you get it out, there will be no wolf to bite you in your living room. If you get the excess glucose out of your body (and make sure it stays out), there will be no excess glucose in your bloodstream to mess up your body organs.

So in what other ways do diabetes drugs harm you? To understand this, we need to look at some simple facts, and see how they add up.

Diabetes drugs operate in different ways and, therefore, to understand why they are bad for you (besides, of course, the fact that they are not curative), we need to look at the different groups of drugs separately.

1. Drugs that increase the production of insulin

Different families of chemicals act to increase the production of insulin by your pancreas. These include sulfonylureas, meglitinides, and phenylalanine derivatives. Besides the critical problems with using drugs of this kind, explained in detail below, sulfonylureas can cause hunger and weight gain, dark-colored urine, upset stomach, and skin reactions.

Meglitinides can cause joint pain, back pain, headache, cold or flu-like symptoms, diarrhea, nausea, and temporary hair loss.

But that is nothing, compared with the long-term damage to your body:

More insulin = more glucose stored in your body cells, unless you keep sugar out of your body. Diabetes medications allow you to eat wrong foods in a guilt-free manner.

Your body needs insulin to store fat. Without insulin, your body is unable to store fat and that's why people who suffer from untreated type 1 diabetes become thin. Their pancreas does not make insulin. Only when they receive insulin artificially do they start to put on weight again.

But excess insulin means more ability to store fat, and when you take this class of diabetes drugs, you produce more insulin. You need to, because of the resistance that your body has developed to insulin, from which it follows that to keep a normal blood glucose level you need more insulin than a healthy person.

Insulin resistance is the result of excess fat in your pancreas and liver. But the greater the insulin resistance you develop, the more insulin you need to keep your blood glucose low and your doctor happy. As a result, you store more fat and increase the resistance to insulin in your body.

So here is the vicious circle that you create when you decide to deal with your diabetes by taking these drugs:

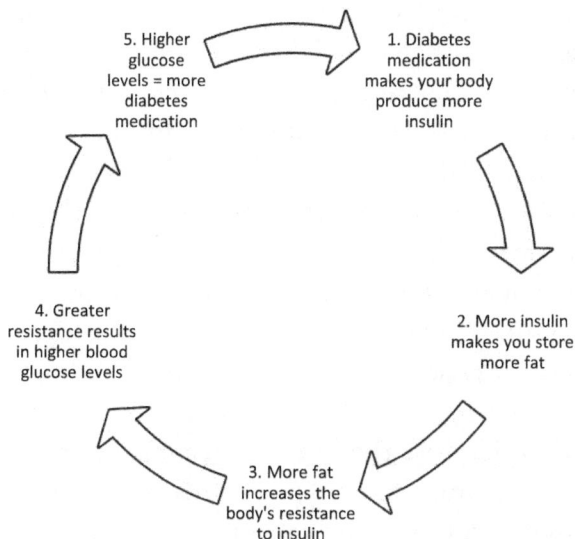

Fig. 4: The Vicious Circle of Diabetes Medication

An important role of insulin is to help store excess energy, which it does in two ways: 1) Glucose molecules can be linked into long chains called glycogen and then stored in the liver. There is, however, a limit to the amount of glycogen that can be stored away. 2) Once the glycogen storage limit is reached, the body starts to turn glucose into fat, by a process called de novo lipogenesis, and stores it in the liver or in fat deposits in the body. Turning glucose into fat is a more complicated process than storing it as glycogen, but there is no limit to the amount of fat that can be created. Obesity follows.

It is therefore clear that taking diabetes medication to increase the production of insulin is a slippery slope that is eventually likely to overwork your pancreas beyond repair, to no useful end other than hiding the disease from view.

2. Drugs that help cells respond more effectively to insulin

The family of drugs known as "TZD" (thiazolidinediones) increases insulin sensitivity and is linked to an increase in the risk of fractures and heart failure. Other side effects include stomach pain, painful urination and/or blood in the urine, shortness of breath, swelling, chest pain, rapid weight gain, and the feeling of being ill. Bad, isn't it?

But besides those side effects, increasing the ability of cells to take more glucose is not the answer. It's like making your basement in our little story bigger, to keep more wolves in. Instead of using more insulin to hide more glucose in our body, it helps us to do it using the existing amount of insulin. Again, not a cure.

3. Drugs that decrease the liver's glucose production

The best-known drug of this type is metformin, which tells the liver to produce less glucose, and/or temporarily suppress the digestive enzymes that turn carbohydrates into glucose, slowing digestion and glucose absorption.

This is a good point to take some time to discuss the central role of the liver. The liver acts as the body's glucose reservoir. Glucose is one of the body fuels and therefore the role of the liver in keeping the circulating blood sugar levels and other body fuels steady and constant is critical. The liver both stores and manufactures glucose according to the body's needs. The way the liver "knows" about the need to store or release glucose is mainly via the hormones insulin and glucagon.

During a meal, the liver stores glucose as glycogen, which will be released when the body needs it. The storage of glucose as glycogen occurs because during a meal the level of insulin is high and that of glucagon is low.

The liver supplies sugar (glucose), when needed, by turning glycogen into glucose in a process called glycogenolysis. The liver can also manufacture glucose by harvesting amino acids, waste products, and fat byproducts, in a process called gluconeogenesis.

Now, what happens when there isn't enough sugar to supply the energy needed by the body? The liver makes another fuel, ketones. Keep an eye on this fuel, because we will be talking about it again in the next chapters.

Some body organs, such as the brain and parts of the kidney, as well as red blood cells, always require sugar. To supplement a limited sugar supply (when there is not enough sugar to meet the demand), the liver makes the alternative fuels ketones, **from fats**, in a process called ketogenesis. The hormone signal for ketogenesis to begin is a low level of insulin. Ketones are burned as fuel by muscles and other body organs. And the sugar is saved for the organs that need it.

Are you starting to see a trend? A low level of insulin equals ketogenesis, which means that our body is burning fat. Less fat means less insulin resistance and, hence, less need for insulin. Yes, now you see it.

4. Other Drugs

In addition to those discussed above, other diabetes drugs are being developed, with more or less severe side effects. But the common characteristic of all diabetes drugs is that they do not cure the diabetes. They keep it at bay, they hide it from view, and in many cases they are a necessity, because the patient lacks the will to get well or is physically unable to do what it takes to reverse his or her diabetes.

Drugs are here to help us when taking them is inevitable, and I don't want to give the impression that one should automatically stop taking diabetes medication. Reversing diabetes is not an easy task. It can be done, but not everybody can do it, simply because it's hard work.

Ignoring the Evidence

The evidence and the strong motivation for reversing type 2 diabetes is clearly and easily available, but the medical profession does not have a hard time ignoring it. An interesting example is the reported effect of bariatric surgery for type 2 diabetes reversal. Bariatric surgery refers to a variety of procedures designed for restricting the passage of food through the stomach. The literature reports long-lasting reversal of diabetes in obese patients after bariatric surgery. The results achieved are quite amazing: around 80% of patients completely reversed their diabetes after bariatric surgery. These results are reported widely in the medical literature and one example is a 2011 review by Andrei Keidar.[50]

These articles offer various hypotheses for this remarkable result, but the most important conclusion to me was a simple one: **Diabetes can be reversed. Period.**

That does not stop people, who cannot be confused by facts, from saying that diabetes cannot be reversed. Even the results published by Newcastle University Professor Roy Taylor, at the European Association for the Study of Diabetes meeting in Lisbon, on September 11, 2017,[51] which conclusively showed that diabetes can be reversed, did not create any noticeable change in the way the medical profession addresses the problem. They keep telling you to shut up, to take your medicine, and to like it.

Professor Taylor's findings can be summarized as follows:

◆ Excess calories lead to excess fat in the liver.

◆ As a result, the liver responds poorly to insulin and produces too much glucose.

◆ Excess fat in the liver is passed on to the pancreas, causing the insulin-producing cells to fail.

---

[50] Diabetes Care 2011 May; 34 (Supplement 2): S361–S266.
https://doi.org/10.2337/dc11-s254
[51]http://www.ncl.ac.uk/press/articles/archive/2017/09/type2diabetesisrevers ible/

◆ Losing less than 1 gram of fat from the pancreas through diet can re-start the normal production of insulin, reversing type 2 diabetes.

◆ This reversal of diabetes remains possible for at least 10 years after the onset of the condition.

Professor Taylor's main conclusion agrees with those of other researchers, who believe that type 2 diabetes actually is caused by excess fat within both the liver and pancreas.

Professor Taylor explains that as insulin controls the normal process of making glucose, the liver then produces too much glucose. Simultaneously, excess fat in the liver increases the normal process of exporting fat to all tissues. In the pancreas, this excess fat causes the insulin-producing cells to fail.

Regardless of whether everybody agrees with the explanation of the mechanism behind it, the important fact remains that losing substantial weight quickly, which removes liver and pancreas fat, results in a reversal of diabetes. That appears to be the result both with bariatric surgery and with the extreme diet used by Professor Taylor in his research.

Takeaways from This Chapter:

It is not hard to see that the way to reverse type 2 diabetes is the exact opposite of what drugs do: In order to reverse your diabetes, you must achieve the following results:

▶ Reduce your body's resistance to insulin.

▶ To do so, you must get rid of the fat that envelops your inner organs.

▶ You cannot get rid of the fat as long as your body produces high amounts of insulin under the influence of your medication.

► It therefore follows that the first thing you must do is to reduce the level of insulin in your body, not to increase it and even not to keep it at its current level—the exact opposite of what your medication is doing.

► Reducing the level of insulin will help you to get rid of the inner fat, which in turn will improve your body's ability to utilize what insulin there is, thus requiring less insulin.

Now you see why your doctor is harming you when he prescribes diabetes medications without first motivating you to discover whether you can reverse your diabetes naturally. He doesn't do it maliciously. In fact, I am sure that every doctor who prescribes diabetes medication is certain that he is doing the right thing for his patient. Only he isn't.

CHAPTER 7
The Doctor–Dietician Collusion

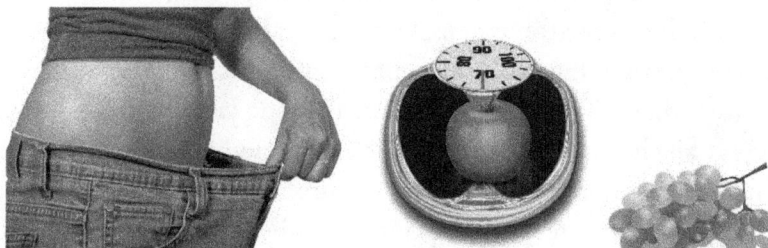

You are what you eat, so it follows that eating right will keep you healthy or will help you to overcome your problem. If you are obese, diabetic, plagued with CD or IBS (or if you have some other food-related condition), your general practitioner may suggest that you consult with a dietician. To me it is obvious (and so it should be to you) that for a dietician (or a nutritionist, as some of them are called) to make a living he cannot give simple, straightforward advice. It has to be complicated, almost mystical, so you will be willing to pay for what you are getting. While I am not suggesting that dieticians are never useful, I will point out examples of how they can be harmful. And since often patients are referred to a dietician by a doctor, as part of the treatment, they have a place in this book.

The profession of dieticians finds its formal roots around the 1950s. As a side comment, it should be noted that before those times obesity was not an epidemic, and diseases associated with wrong eating were not that common. Sure, a few obese people existed, but that was not a widespread problem. So, one wonders, why do we need a dietician to tell us to eat moderately and to limit ourselves to healthy food as we did before?

To illustrate the point let's consider again the advice you are receiving if you have been diagnosed with type 2 diabetes. There is wide agreement that diabetics must watch their weight and since they are usually overweight, they must lose as much as needed to get back to a normal body mass index (BMI). The question then becomes, how can you go about losing weight easily and effectively? Even after you make the courageous decision to go on a diet, you are misled by the many (more or less) authoritative sources that tell you that if you are diabetic you must make sure to eat all the time. If you listen to idiotic advice from so-called "nutrition experts," you will make sure never to be hungry. The fibs that are shouted at you from everywhere are that you have to maintain a constant eating regime, never to miss a single meal, or else your blood sugar will spiral out of control. You will be given complicated menus, the only effect of which is to keep you busy and worried all day long, and since they are sometimes difficult to follow, they are sure to make you feel inadequate and a failure. As explained in Chapter 6, because the net result of the suggested dietary regimes is inevitably a continuously high level of insulin during the day, it results in more weight gain.

You will find well-meaning sources of information on diabetes telling you that "... regularly scheduled meals and snacks are best for glycemic control. This is a long-well-known principle."[52] Even respected medical sources, like the Mayo Clinic,

---

[52] https://www.thediabetescouncil.com/does-timing-of-food-matter-with-diabetes/

will give you similar directions.[53] The following, for instance, is what the clinic proposes that you should eat if you are diabetic:

"**Breakfast.** Whole-wheat bread (1 medium slice) with 2 teaspoons jelly, 1/2 cup shredded wheat cereal with a cup of 1 percent low-fat milk, a piece of fruit, coffee

Lunch. Cheese and veggie pita, medium apple with 2 tablespoons almond butter, water

Dinner. Salmon, 1 1/2 teaspoons vegetable oil, small baked potato, 1/2 cup carrots, side salad (1 1/2 cups spinach, 1/2 of a tomato, 1/4 cup chopped bell pepper, 2 teaspoons olive oil, 1 1/2 teaspoons red wine vinegar), unsweetened iced tea

Snack. 2 1/2 cups popcorn or an orange with 1/2 cup 1 percent low-fat cottage cheese"

This means that you will be constantly eating during the day. Moreover, you will be eating a lot of carbs, which goes against every logic I can think of. Whole-wheat bread, wheat cereal, fruit, baked potatoes, carrots, tomatoes, and popcorn are all carbohydrate bombs, so one wonders what the clinic was thinking when suggesting that diet. But of course, if the dietician who concocted that advice told you "stop eating all the time and stay away from carbs," you might have felt that you were not getting value for your money. "It has to be more sophisticated and complicated than that," could be your instinctive reaction. Well, it doesn't (and as we learned in Chapter 5, our instincts are often wrong).

Most diets are designed to keep the wolves in the basement (i.e., the sugar in the cells). You will find hundreds of such

---

[53] https://www.mayoclinic.org/diseases-conditions/diabetes/in-depth/diabetes-diet/art-20044295

suggestions on the web, making what I now understand are foolish statements, such as:[54]

"Generally, it is recommended to eat breakfast within 90 minutes of waking and then eat at least every 4–5 hours during the day after your first meal. Snacks are not necessary, but can be included if hunger is present between meals. In fact, bedtime snacks are very helpful. Since it is recommended to avoid going more than 10 hours overnight without eating, a bedtime snack containing 15–30 grams of carbohydrates, combined with a low-fat protein, prevents the liver from releasing extra, stored glucose into the bloodstream and assists in the management of fasting blood sugars."

A detailed discussion of what you should be doing instead, if you have type 2 diabetes, exceeds the scope of this book and can be found elsewhere.[55] This condition is a great example of a cascade of misconceptions and wrong medical and dietary advice, so I have used it to make the point. However, since we are talking about losing weight, if you have a condition that requires it, I recommend reading Doctor Jason Fung's *The Complete Guide to Fasting*,[56] which contains greatly useful information in an easily readable form. If reading the whole book is too much for you, you can still find extremely useful information on Doctor Fung's blog.[57]

---

[54] https://foodandnutrition.org/blogs/stone-soup/meal-times-diabetes-whats-connection/
[55] Luzzatto, Kfir. *How to Reverse Your Diabetes (If You Really Mean It).*
[56] Fung, Jason, & Moore, Jimmy. *The Complete Guide to Fasting: Heal Your Body Through Intermittent, Alternate-Day, and Extended.* Victory Belt Publishing
[57] https://www.dietdoctor.com/intermittent-fasting/questions-and-answers

What Happens When We Fast?

Insulin levels drop and the body starts to burn stored energy. Glycogen (the glucose that's stored in the liver) can provide energy for approximately 24 hours. After that, the body starts to break down stored body fat for energy. If we continue to eat throughout the day as the experts would have us do, we will gain weight. To avoid weight gain and to promote weight loss, we need to increase the amount of time we burn food energy, by fasting. In the context of this discussion, "fasting" simply means that we are not eating (not that we are doing anything special).

Fasting results in low insulin levels, which stimulate lipolysis, the breakdown of fat for energy. Although the brain uses glucose as fuel, it can also use ketone bodies, which are generated during fasting (and also in a keto diet). In prolonged fasting (more than four days), about 75% of the energy used by the brain is provided by ketones. The process also leads to high levels of growth hormone, which maintain muscle mass and lean tissues.[58] So what happens is that the body switches naturally from burning glucose to burning fat, which is the body's stored food energy. There is no undesirable effect on other tissues: the body does not "burn muscle" in an effort to feed itself; the increased levels of growth hormone see to that.

There are several different ways to fast, and you must choose the one that works for you. Obese people who need to slim quickly may fast for days in a row. On the light side, you have the 20-hour fast, in which you only eat in a four-hour window once a day, and the 16-hour fast, in which in addition you also have a light meal 16 hours after the last one. More extended fasts can last for 32 hours up to several weeks. At first, when teaching your body to fast, you may want to adopt different fasting schedules, but in the end you will need to come up with something that

---

[58] http://diabetes.diabetesjournals.org/content/50/1/96

integrates well with your day. The beauty of this method is that you can find a schedule that works for you without upsetting your daily routine. Once you reach your target weight you will find a routine that maintains it, which will likely be lighter than the one you adopted at first, when you needed to shed a lot of weight.

And guess what: intermittent fasting can be an alternative to many other treatments (notably, bariatric surgery for obese patients, which exposes patients to severe risks). But no dietician will recommend it to you, nor will the majority of physicians. Imagine them telling you "You don't need me at all. Just take up intermittent fasting." It doesn't look likely that this will happen any time soon.

You cannot compare the complex diets that the experts propose with fasting. For one thing, fasting is very easy and simple: instead of worrying all the time about what you will be eating in your next eating window, you simply skip it. It doesn't get any simpler than that. Intermittent fasting is not some extraordinary way of living, but rather it represents going back to the way in which human beings have been eating for millennia. We have been conditioned for decades by the food industry to consume, eat, and stuff ourselves with processed foods as many times during the day as they managed to convince us to do. We need to take a step back and understand that we must stop being a willing target of those who want to sell us snacks and other processed foods for the sole purpose of making a profit. We must switch back to eating when it's good for us, when we need it, and when our body really wants it.

And this brings me back to my beef with the medical system (which, as said, includes dietologists of all kinds—although this may not actually be a proper word). That people who make a living by selling unhealthy processed foods to other people will do their utmost to convince us to buy those foods is understandable, if not commendable. But that the medical profession has allowed itself to become a choir that sings to the tune of that industry is, in my opinion, inexcusable.

Doctors on Autopilot

A dear and close relative of mine was well over 90 years old and had been twice already in the clutches of Death, out of which he had rather miraculously managed to pull himself. In spite of his surprising survival, he was in very bad shape, prey to dementia and unable to care for himself. He was barely able to communicate with people around him, and even that only at times. I happened to be near him during one of the routine visits of his doctor. To pass the time I glanced at the endless list of medicines that he was taking daily, and something grabbed my attention.

"Why is he taking statins?" I asked the doctor.

"His cholesterol is high. He needs statins," the doctor answered.

"But at his age and the conditions he is in, that would be the least of his problems, wouldn't it?" I pointed out.

"Perhaps, but that's what should be prescribed with the cholesterol levels that he has," the doctor said, obviously considering the argument closed.

This is a good example of the knee-jerk reactions that many doctors have to a blood test. The statins prescription is also invariably followed by stern instructions to avoid meat, fat, and pretty much everything else you like. As I tried to convince a doctor friend of mine in a similar context, it may perhaps be considered by some as a measure that helps you to live longer, but it makes living no longer worthwhile. In the case of uselessly cruel dietary restrictions, of course, it does not make you healthier, only sadder.

A great discussion of this topic can be found in the excellent book *The Great Cholesterol Myth*,[59] which is written in a form clearly readable by the general public, but still supported with well-explained science. Among many other interesting things that one can learn from it are the following:

> *Cholesterol is a relatively minor player in heart disease and a poor predictor of heart attacks. More than half of all people who are hospitalized with heart attacks have perfectly normal cholesterol levels.*

and:

> *Saturated fat has been wrongfully demonized. Saturated fat raises "good" (HDL) cholesterol. Saturated fat tends to change the pattern of your "bad" (LDL) cholesterol to the more favorable pattern A (big, fluffy particles). Several recent studies have shown that saturated fat is not associated with a greater risk of heart disease. One study from Harvard concluded that "greater saturated fat intake is associated with less progression of coronary atherosclerosis, whereas carbohydrate intake is associated with a greater progression."*

and finally:

> *Statins should not be prescribed for the elderly or for the vast majority of women, and they should never be prescribed for children. Research shows that (with rare exceptions) any benefit from statin drugs is seen only*

---

[59] Bowden, Jonny. *The Great Cholesterol Myth + 100 Recipes for Preventing and Reversing Heart Disease*. Fair Winds Press.

in middle-aged men with documented coronary artery disease.

To your average dietician, all the above is heresy and you should be burned at the stake for merely considering it. However, the evidence in favor of these conclusions is compelling, and it makes all the dietary advice that we know look silly. Of course, you must consider your particular situation and make up your own mind as to what you want to do about your cholesterol. But before you do, please read the available literature and *then* make up your mind. You shouldn't care if your doctor operates on autopilot and has a Pavlovian reflex that makes him or her reach for the statin prescription every time they see a certain cholesterol value in your blood test. You need to weigh the pros and cons (including side effects such as the increased danger of becoming diabetic or of losing your sex drive if you take statins). Once again, if you need your medicine, you must make peace with its side effects; but if you don't, there is no excuse for you to endure them.

Takeaways from This Chapter:

▶ Diets often have the effect of complicating your day with little or no positive results. In fact, wrong dietary advice, which is not uncommon, may do much more harm than not dieting.
▶ Fasting may have better and faster results than complex diets for conditions in which it is appropriate, but dieticians will not suggest it to you.
▶ Some doctors will prescribe a treatment to you based on tests results, which is commonly accepted but may be wrong for you (doctors on autopilot).

CHAPTER 8
"Have Scalpel, Will Operate"

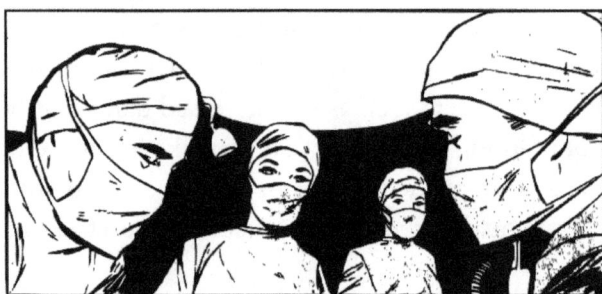

Let's be realistic: Surgeons want to cut you open. They have no interest in sending you home with a pill and a pat on the back, because that's not what they have been trained to do. They have been taught to fix things with brute force, pretty much like a plumber or a carpenter. Their education conditions them to find what's wrong with you, and if it can be fixed by cutting you up, they'll fix it. And then, there is that little matter of the money ...

A study[60] examined surgical procedures carried out in the period 2008–2016, and you may want to sit down to read the results of that analysis:

---

[60] https://www.ncbi.nlm.nih.gov/pmc/articles/PMC5735893/pdf/ 13037_2017_Article_144.pdf

Unnecessary procedures were performed for at least five years in most cases (53.2%); 56.3% of the cases involved 30 or more patients, and 37.5% involved 100 or more patients. In nearly all cases the physician was male (96.2%) and working in private practice (92.4%); 57.0% of the physicians had an accomplice, 48.1% were 50 years of age or older, and 40.5% trained outside the U.S. The most common motives were financial gain (92.4%) and suspected antisocial personality (48.1%), followed by poor problem-solving or clinical skills (11.4%) and ambition (3.8%). The most common environmental factors that provided opportunity for unnecessary procedures included a lack of oversight (40.5%) or oversight failures (39.2%), a corrupt moral climate (26.6%), vulnerable patients (20.3%), and financial conflicts of interest (13.9%).

Scary, isn't it?

It is not that I want to rub it in, but I do want you to be shaken, horrified, and sensitized, because what this review tells us goes head-on against everything we expect from physicians, and we need to bring our expectations to a more realistic level. So here are some specific details of the finding of that analysis:

A Louisiana physician performed unnecessary cardiac catheterizations and stents, angiograms, and angioplasties on approximately 310 patients over at least 5 years; one patient died and hundreds of others suffered harm. A Florida ophthalmologist misdiagnosed patients with wet macular degeneration to justify unnecessary laser eye surgery. He falsified patient records and ordered unnecessary diagnostic tests to support his fabricated diagnoses. A South Dakota surgeon repeatedly performed medically unnecessary spinal surgeries for profit, resulting in patient injury and death. Despite complaints filed by his medical staff and former patients and their family members, he retained his privileges and continued to practice for many years.

So now you know why you have to doubt your doctor and develop your own skills, to help you to emerge unscathed from a medical adventure.

Useless Surgery Never Stops

The American Medical Association (AMA) claimed that *"2.4 million unnecessary operations were performed on Americans at a cost of $3.9 billion and that 11,900 patients had died from unneeded operations (...)"*. But wait, that was in 1976! So by now that must have stopped, you will think. Well, think again. One well-known example of useless surgery is the spinal fusion for back pain. If you Googled it at the time of writing this book (in mid-2018), you found "about 19,400,000 results," many of which do not highlight to you the uselessness of the procedure, but, quite the contrary, make it look sophisticated and appealing. Take for example the list of medical conditions that this procedure addresses, according to a reputable medical institute (let's call it "Clinic" for convenience):

> **Broken vertebrae.** *Not all broken vertebrae require spinal fusion. Many heal without treatment. But if a broken vertebra makes your spinal column unstable, spinal fusion surgery may be necessary.*
>
> **Deformities of the spine.** *Spinal fusion can help correct spinal deformities, such as a sideways curvature of the spine (scoliosis) or abnormal rounding of the upper spine (kyphosis).*
>
> **Spinal weakness or instability.** *Your spine may become unstable if there's abnormal or excessive motion between two vertebrae. This is a common side effect of severe arthritis in the spine. Spinal fusion can be used to restore spinal stability in such cases.*

Spondylolisthesis. In this spinal disorder, one vertebra slips forward and onto the vertebra below it. Spinal fusion may be needed to treat spondylolisthesis if the condition causes severe back pain or nerve crowding that produces leg pain or numbness.

Herniated disk. Spinal fusion may be used to stabilize the spine after removal of a damaged (herniated) disk.

In all fairness, it must be said that Clinic also recognizes that risks exist. Unfortunately, it does so in these words: *"Spinal fusion is generally a safe procedure. But as with any surgery, spinal fusion carries the potential risk of complications."*

So what is the first thing we learn from this sentence that Clinic puts there to tell us about the risks of this surgery? That **Spinal fusion is generally a safe procedure!** Well, now that we know that, we can stop worrying, and that's the starting point from which we will look at any further information given us. That's the power of framing. What a pity for Clinic that 31 of the world's leading back pain researchers have published a call to action in the authoritative medical journal *The Lancet*, saying that lower back pain is being mistreated on an enormous scale.[61] According to them, for instance, *"Hundreds of thousands of Australian back pain sufferers are being given harmful or useless treatments."*

Of course, if we belong to that annoying group of nosy patients that some doctors hate so much, who will go on reading what Clinic tells us about this procedure, we will be finally relieved of our doubts when we read what we can expect after the surgery: *"A hospital stay of two to three days is usually required following spinal fusion. Depending on the location and extent of*

---

[61] https://www.smh.com.au/national/thousands-of-back-pain-sufferers-given-harmful-treatments-20180321-p4z5h0.html

your surgery, you may experience some pain and discomfort but the pain can usually be well-controlled with medications."

What are we waiting for? Two or three days of hospital stay with well-controlled pain is barely worse than a visit to the dentist. But let's look at the "warning" that the potential complications listed include: *"infection, poor wound healing, bleeding, blood clots, injury to blood vessels or nerves in and around the spine, and pain at the site from which the bone graft is taken."* None of that sounds particularly ominous, however, since in every surgery similar "minor" complications can be expected (and by the time we read it we have been conditioned to think of them as "unlikely," at least for us). However, the University of Maryland Medical Center has a different take on the complications of spinal surgery.[62] According to its patient's guide, the following unpleasant additional complications may occur (in addition to those encountered with every surgery, such as anesthesia and blood clot complications):

Hardware Fracture – In many different types of spinal operations, metal screws, plates, and rods are used as part of the procedure to hold the vertebrae in alignment while the surgery heals. These metal devices are called "hardware." ... Sometimes before the surgery is completely healed the hardware can either break – or move from the correct position. This is called a "hardware fracture." If this occurs it may require a second operation to either remove the hardware or replace the hardware.

Implant Migration – Implant migration is a term used to describe the fact that the implant has moved from where the surgeon placed it initially ... If the implant moves too far, it may

---

[62] https://www.umms.org/ummc/health-services/orthopedics/services/spine/patient-guides/complications-spine-surgery

not be doing its job of stabilizing the two vertebrae. If it moves in a direction towards the spine or large vessels – it may damage those structures.

Spinal Cord Injury *– Any time you operate on the spine, there is some risk of injuring the spinal cord ... Damage to the spinal cord can cause paralysis in certain areas and not others, depending on which spinal nerves are affected.*

Persistent Pain *– ... One of the most common complications of spinal surgery is that it does not get rid of all of your pain. In some cases, it may be possible to actually increase your pain.*

Sexual Dysfunction *– ... Damage to the spinal cord and the nerves around the spinal cord can cause many problems. If a nerve is damaged that connects to the pelvic region, it could cause sexual dysfunction.*

Transitional Syndrome *– ... if one or more levels are fused anywhere in the spine, the spinal segment next to where the surgery was performed begins to take on more stress. Over time, this can lead to increased wear and tear to this segment, eventually causing pain from the damaged segment.*

Pseudoarthrosis *– ... When the vertebrae involved in a surgical fusion do not heal and fuse together, there is usually continued pain. The pain may actually increase over time.*

So now that you have read these explanations, how do you feel about spinal fusion surgery? Compare with how you felt after reading the explanations that the Clinic supplied, and you will have another good example of framing.

Not Just the Spine

Because I concentrated on the broadly advertised and ill-reputed spinal fusion surgery, I don't want the reader to think that it is the only problematic surgery. Examples abound in which physical therapy does the same (and better) than surgery, with fewer risks and less discomfort. For example, another common surgery for pain management is that for a meniscal tear and osteoarthritis. A recent study[63] found that physical therapy was as effective long term as surgery, in 70% of the patients studied (30% of the patients in the physical therapy group elected to have surgery for whatever reason). That's a huge find. In humanly understandable terms, at least 70 out of 100 people who were sent to surgery could have happily fixed their problem by doing the right physical exercise. Consider that figure again: 70 out of 100.

Pete Egoscue's Method

I have become a Pete Egoscue disciple. I spread the word about his teachings and buy his book[64] as a present to people I care about. Why? Because it works. I have experienced it personally, and I have seen it work with others. His basic theory is simple: Being truly pain free depends on rediscovery, not reengineering. By rediscovering the body's design and allowing it to work as intended, many of the disabling conditions that take a financial and personal toll can be reversed or avoided altogether.

Dealing with pain requires understanding its source and then acting upon that understanding, instead of going to someone who will fix it for us. I am citing below Egoscue's explanation of knee surgery, because it is so revealing:

---

[63] https://www.nejm.org/doi/10.1056/NEJMoa1301408
[64] Egoscue, Pete. *Pain Free: A Revolutionary Method for Stopping Chronic Pain.*

Since knees are damaged more than any other joint, a whole industry has developed to service them and eliminate pain. Knee surgery is the Midas muffler of orthopedics. Repair the joint—or replace it—and move on. Physicians, being human, are not immune to buying into the assumptions that the rest of us make. We go to doctors to relieve pain, they oblige us, then they see the next patient. Gradually, they lose track of the cause-and-effect relationship because the effect—chronic musculoskeletal pain— returns in different forms accompanied by different symptomatic events, or "causes." Instead of skiing, the victim was playing squash, and he or she smashed up a shoulder. The logical circle has been broken. The doctor dutifully fixes the shoulder and never makes the connection between the two episodes because accidents happen. Besides, knees are fragile. Almost every client who comes to my clinic is a refugee from this crazed geometric progression that starts with a minor dysfunctional condition and carries on from symptomatic event to symptomatic event right to the brink of catastrophe.

You owe it to yourself to explore every existing natural solution to your pain, before climbing on that operation table and submitting yourself to the scalpel.

Doctors Speak Up

There is little doubt that your average surgeon is wired for ... surgery. He is not "scalpel happy"—it's what he has been taught to do and why he exists in the medical system. His job is not to tell you to go home and do some Pilates.

Lately, however, some doctors have spoken up, and that shows you how big the problem is. It is instructive to read the editorial[65] by Philip F. Stahel, Todd F. VanderHeiden, and Fernando J. Kim, which asks *"Why do surgeons continue to*

---

[65] https://www.ncbi.nlm.nih.gov/pmc/articles/PMC5234149

perform unnecessary surgery?" The answer is quite chilling, so I report it here *verbatim*:

> *From a surgeon's perspective, two distinct answers appear intuitive:*
> *1. We perform surgery because we have been trained to do so and because "we have always done it this way" or we simply do not know any better. In German psychology, this behavior is analogous to a historic entity termed "Funktionslust."*
> *2. We are incentivized to perform surgical procedures, either for financial gain, renown, or both.*

Takeaways from This Chapter:

▶ Unnecessary invasive procedures (such as surgery) are a reality. One must always take into account the possibility that a proposed invasive treatment is useless and, often, harmful.

▶ Medical institutes that make large profits from useless surgery will frame the procedure and its dangers in a way that makes them desirable, while making sure to mention all the dangers so as to be able to argue that the patient has received a full disclosure.

▶ Where the problem has to do with orthopedic problems, physical therapy is in many cases an effective, non-invasive solution that should be explored before agreeing to surgery.

CHAPTER 9
Useless (and Dangerous) Testing

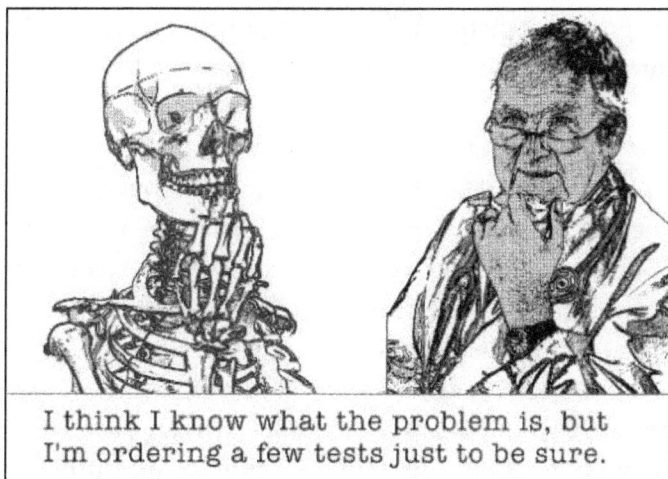

I think I know what the problem is, but I'm ordering a few tests just to be sure.

Sometimes doctors are a bit like children—they like to play with their toys. They have these big, new, shiny machines that spit out cool images or graphs and numbers that only they can decipher, and they want to put you into them and play. And then, they are scared—and rightly so—that if it turns out that you have a condition that could have been detected by one of those toys and they didn't use it, they may be accused of malpractice. A 2017 research on overtreatment in America[66] found that in 84.7% of the cases the most commonly cited reasons for overtreatment concerned fear of malpractice. So why not run a few more tests so that, if something goes wrong with the patient, we will be able to show that we were not negligent? After all, it is not the referring physician who operates the machines, and it's no hassle at all to order a battery of tests (and the more sophisticated, the better) and to send you away feeling that you are getting value for your money. But are you?

Forget the gut-wrenching feeling that you will have before, during, and after the test, until the results are explained to you, with the associated stress that, in itself, is bad for your health. Forget also the cost to the system, which will eventually come out of your pockets, whether you know it or not. The real problem is that some of those tests may be directly harmful.

What is "Medical Overuse"?

Overuse is defined as the provision of medical services for which the potential for harm exceeds the potential for benefit, a problem that is increasingly recognized around the world. According to an article published in the authoritative medical journal *Lancet*,[67] in the United States, estimates of spending on overuse vary widely: conservative estimates based on direct measurement of individual services range from 6% to 8% of total health care spending, while studies of geographic variation (an indirect measure) put the proportion of Medicare spending on overuse closer to 29%. Around the world, overuse of some individual services may be as high as 80% of cases. While overuse has been best documented in high-income countries (HICs), low- and middle-income

[66] https://www.ncbi.nlm.nih.gov/pmc/articles/PMC5587107/pdf/pone.0181970.pdf
[67] https://www.ncbi.nlm.nih.gov/pmc/articles/PMC5708862/pdf/nihms897023.pdf

countries (LMICs) are not immune, and evidence suggestive of widespread overuse is accumulating from countries and health systems as diverse as Australia, Spain, Israel, Brazil, and Iran. Overuse can coexist with unmet health needs, particularly in LMICs. The authors address specifically the issue of overuse of diagnostic tests:

> *Overuse of testing appears to be common, driven by availability, apparent objectiveness, and the increasing sensitivity of tests to detect disease. Despite few systematic analyses of inappropriate use of diagnostic tests in general, some specific diagnostic services have been evaluated around the world. Overuse of endoscopy, for instance, appears to be common globally. In primary care practices in Switzerland, 14% of colonoscopy referrals and 49% of referrals for upper endoscopy represented overuse. Elsewhere in Europe, appropriateness rates for endoscopy have been reported in Portugal, Spain, Italy, and Norway, with overuse accounting for between 13% and 33% of tests, and at an Israeli center 16% of endoscopies were unnecessary. Studies in the US have reported overuse rates as high as 60%.*

So whatever the statistics that fit your case, you are at high risk of being referred to a test that you don't need and that can harm you.

There are, however, some areas in which screening is low risk and has a high benefit, in which giving up the option of being screened would plainly be irresponsible. An important example is screening of newborns, as discussed in a 2016 article published in *The Journal of Law, Medicine & Ethics.*[68] The purpose of this chapter is not to turn you into an indiscriminate enemy of screening, but rather to show you that while in some cases

---

[68] https://www.ncbi.nlm.nih.gov/pmc/articles/PMC5381153/pdf/nihms853525.pdf

screening is very important and may be life-saving, in others it may be useless and even dangerous. Like everywhere else in this book, the message is that you cannot abdicate the responsibility to your health by taking a recommendation from your doctor as if it were automatically worth following.

Negative Example:
Mammography for Breast Cancer Screening

The equipment used to perform mammography has become increasingly sensitive and can now detect extremely small tumors, which would not be found otherwise. That means that you can operate on those tiny tumors and get rid of them before they have a chance to grow and become really dangerous. So the equipment allows to perform preventive surgery while the tumor is still in its initial stages. That's great, right? **Wrong!**

A study published in the *Lancet Oncology Journal* in 2011[69] illustrates this point. The authors compared cumulative breast cancer incidence in age-matched cohorts of women living in seven Swedish counties before and after the initiation of public mammography screening between 1986 and 1990. Women aged 40–49 years were invited to screening every year and women aged 50–74 years were invited every 2 years. A screened group including 328,927 women aged 40–69 years was followed-up for 6 years after the first invitation to the program. A control group including 317,404 women in the same age range was also followed-up for 6 years—4 years without screening and 2 years when they entered the screening program. Screening attendance was much the same in both groups (close to 80%). The findings of this extensive review including a large number of women were troubling: Before the age-matched controls were invited to be screened at the end of their follow-up period, the 4-year

---

[69] http://www.breastcancerchoices.org/files/swedishmammo2011.pdf

cumulative incidence of invasive breast cancer was significantly higher in the screened group (982 per 100,000) than it was in the control group (658 per 100,000). Even after prevalence screening in the control group, the screened group had a higher 6-year cumulative incidence of invasive breast cancer. The only conclusion that the authors could draw from the facts was *"that many invasive breast cancers detected by repeated mammography screening do not persist to be detected by screening at the end of 6 years, suggesting that the natural course of many of the screen-detected invasive breast cancers is to spontaneously regress."*

As we discussed before, in order to understand the real meaning of what we read we must translate it into real people numbers. Put into plain English, what the study tells us is that in the group that was screened, 1,065 women were told that they had breast cancer, when they didn't. Left alone, the tiny tumors detected in the screening would have gone away and those 1,095 women would have gone on happy with their lives, instead of having surgery and other cancer treatments inflicted on them, and the quality of their lives destroyed forever.

Spontaneous tumor regression is not a fairy tale but a very well-known occurrence in a variety of cancers, as discussed in a 2016 review published in the *Journal of Oncological Sciences.*[70] This follows an article in *Current Oncology,*[71] which concludes that *"Epidemiologic observations in two fields of study lead to the same conclusion: namely, that a proportion of breast cancers will go away without medical or surgical intervention,"* and *"for every 100 nonpalpable cancers found through mammography alone, 54 would presumably have gone away."*

---

[70] https://doi.org/10.1016/j.jons.2016.04.008

[71] http://www.current-oncology.com/index.php/oncology/article/view/1037/845

But, of course, 46 of those cancers were real, and detecting them early means a better chance of recovering. So here is how we should phrase the question:

Do you prefer a 46% chance that if you have a real cancer that must be treated, it will be discovered early, or a 54% chance to be spared becoming a cancer patient, with all it implies, while in fact you are perfectly healthy and what was found in the screening will go away on its own?

That is a tough call if there ever was one. But to make an informed decision you need some more data. While the jury is still out on it, a 2014 review[72] of available data concludes that *"mammography screening in women aged 40–49 years ... did not prove its efficacy in decreasing mortality."* Other research it mentions also points out that annual screening may result in radiation-induced cancers and in deaths from this type of cancer. In other words, there is no free lunch. Screening if you are at risk may be a wise decision, but otherwise you may be putting yourself at risk needlessly.

I am surely not advocating against testing yourself when it makes sense to do so, but the evidence for overscreening and overtesting is compelling, and what it tells us is that you should not go and be screened without weighing the pros and cons, just because someone told you to do it, or because everybody else does it.

Here, again, your body has much to tell you and will signal to you in many cases when something is wrong. Unfortunately, we have a tendency to ignore those signals and to defer testing until we can no longer ignore them, and that's a big mistake, because

---

[72] https://www.ncbi.nlm.nih.gov/pmc/articles/PMC4285825/

that is the time to listen to what your body is saying. An old-school surgeon I knew used to tell me to avoid getting tested as long as I felt fine, but at the first sign that something might be different from usual, to go and get checked without procrastinating. I always found this advice to be wise. That, of course, did not include taking routine blood tests a couple of times a year, which is harmless and can give you a heads up that something isn't as it should before you otherwise notice it.

Positive Example:
Screening for Congenital Hypothyroidism

According to the European Society for Paediatric Endocrinology,[73] about 1 in 2000 to 3000 newborns exhibits Congenital Hypothyroidism (CH)—a condition in which an insufficient level of thyroid hormone is produced. This is a serious condition, because thyroid hormones play a crucial role in early neurodevelopment so that untreated severe CH results in neurological and psychiatric deficits, including intellectual disability, spasticity, and disturbances of gait and co-ordination. CH is one of the most common preventable causes of mental retardation. Screening programs, which have been in operation over the last 30 years in most industrialized countries, have led to the successful early detection and treatment of infants with CH and have eliminated the severe neurodevelopmental deficits resulting from late diagnosis. Studies on cognitive function in patients with CH treated soon after birth have shown that normal development can be achieved in most patients.

Screening for CH is done simply by taking a blood sample (which is taken from newborns anyway), and the treatment, if a deficiency is detected, consists of thyroid hormone replacement, which is safe and simple to administer. Given the dire

---

[73] https://academic.oup.com/jcem/article/99/2/363/2536748

consequences of leaving this condition untreated, the relatively high incidence of the problem (1 in 2000 to 3000 newborns) and the simple and safe treatment of the deficiency, not screening for CH is simply madness.

I wanted to bring up this diametrically opposed example, to show you the flip side. Most parents of newborn babies don't even know that their child has been screened for CH, because no problem was found. So how do you know if your baby was tested? If you live in a modern, industrialized country, chances are that this screening is standard procedure in the hospital where your baby was born. But what if you happen to be temporarily residing in a less-developed country? And what if for whatever reason a mistake was made and your baby's blood was not sent for that test? Knowing everything you need to keep yourself and your family safe through the medical system is daunting, but you don't need to be an expert on everything from birth to old age. You just need to be able to ask the right questions at the appropriate time. The survival kit discussed in Chapter 11 may be of some slight help in crafting your questions. You may be surprised to see that raising a hypothesis or asking whether a specific test has been considered, may change the way your doctor approaches the situation. This has to do with the operation of System 1 and System 2, discussed in Chapter 1. If a simple route is proposed to the doctor's mind, which does not take into account a more complex situation, asking him questions may bring System 2 into action and result in a less simplistic answer that may require additional or alternative testing.

Negative Example:
Screening for Prostate Cancer

For years I have been told that taking a PSA test is important ("PSA" stands for Prostate-Specific Antibody). The early detection of prostate cancer is critical to patient survival, so the test was a standard one for a long time. Each time you take the test you may become the victim of a false positive result with all the negative outcome that this implies, but if it may improve your chances of survival, the risk might be worth taking. But guess what, it doesn't.

A 2015 review[74] found that *"There was no evidence of a prostate cancer mortality reduction in the American PLCO[75] trial, which investigated a screening program in a setting where opportunistic screening was already common practice."* It was little surprise, therefore, when my health provider stopped prescribing the PSA test. Reducing mortality is the ultimate goal, and if screening doesn't do it, it has no reason to be.

One could argue that as long as you give blood anyway there is no reason not to run as many tests on it as available, but that would overlook the test-induced stress on the patient, the additional tests that may have to be taken if false-positive results are received, and the potentially unnecessary invasive procedures that may result.

RUN (Repeat Until Normal)

I mentioned my old family physician's motto before. It is of course not applicable to every situation, because in many cases a test result conclusively indicates that a problem may exist. However:

- Test results may come out wrong because of a machine malfunctioning or if the sample has not been properly handled. For instance, a urine sample that has not been properly kept may return a result indicating an infection of the urinary tract, while

---

[74] https://www.ncbi.nlm.nih.gov/pmc/articles/PMC4561549/pdf/ohtas-15-1.pdf

[75] PLCO is the "Prostate, Lung, Colorectal, and Ovarian Cancer Screening Trial."

none exists and the sample was contaminated at some point along the road.

- You may have contracted a viral infection without knowing it, which will pass soon and with it some irregular test result.

- And finally, our body is a very complex machine and sometimes it needs time to recover from whatever has caused a shift in its behavior, be it food, medicine taken for other reasons, or anything else that affected its behavior.

In all those cases, a repeat test may show that the first result was wrong or indicative of a passing condition. While it is of course not practical or needed to repeat each test every time, when the test results have substantial consequences, such as they indicate that serious therapy should be initiated, discussing repeating the tests with your physician before starting to act on them, is a good policy (see A Real Life Example in Chapter 3).

Takeaways from This Chapter:

▶ In some cases the potential for harm of a medical service exceeds the potential for benefit. This is called "medical overuse."

▶ Medical testing is often overused. Some tests have a potential for harmful results, such as by subjecting the patient to unnecessary therapies.

▶ Nevertheless, in many cases screening for a condition may be extremely important. The patient must take an active role in the decision regarding potential testing.

CHAPTER 10
When Your Doctor Makes You Sick

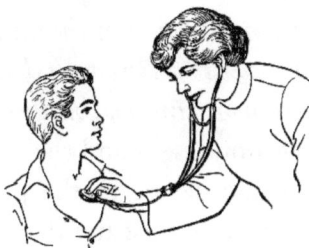

In the dialect of my native city of Milan, Italy, there is a saying that freely translates into: "You may be courting a loss just by looking at this person's face." This applies well to some doctors who are responsible for the well-known nocebo effect, which, simply put, means that you are influenced by the behavior (or even only by the presence) of your doctor. The most innocuous (if troubling) example is the so-called "white coat effect,"[76] which refers to the white coats traditionally worn by doctors. The white coat effect means that your blood pressure is higher when it is taken in a medical setting than it is when taken at home. White coat effects

---

[76] https://www.ahajournals.org/doi/10.1161/HYPERTENSIONAHA.113.01275

will often happen because you are nervous about having your blood pressure tested by a doctor or nurse.

Jo Marchand[77] points out that while warning patients about pain or discomfort that they are about to feel is a staple of conventional medical care, during medical procedures such as scans or operations, we are particularly susceptible to the nocebo effect, and that being told how much things are about to hurt simply worsens our pain. Bruce Lipton,[78] an expert in the biologic effects of our thought, says that *"In medicine, the nocebo effect can be as powerful as the placebo effect, a fact you should keep in mind every time you step into a doctor's office. By their words and their demeanor, physicians can convey hope-deflating messages to their patients, messages that are, I believe, completely unwarranted. ... Another example is the potential power of the statement: 'You have six months to live.' If you choose to believe your doctor's message, you are not likely to have much more time on this Earth."*

The nocebo effect is omnipresent and the reader is certain to have experienced it to some degree in the past. The medical literature also recognizes the existence and the importance of the effect, as seen for instance in a 2012 review by W. Häuser, E. Hansen, and P. Enck,[79] which explains:

> *By definition, a nocebo effect is the induction of a symptom perceived as negative by sham treatment and/or by the suggestion of negative expectations. A nocebo response is a negative symptom induced by the patient's own negative expectations and/or by negative suggestions from clinical staff in the absence of any treatment. The underlying mechanisms include learning by Pavlovian conditioning and reaction to expectations induced by*

---

[77] Marchant, Jo. *Cure: A Journey into the Science of Mind Over Body* (pp. 124–125).
[78] Lipton Ph.D., Bruce H. *The Biology of Belief.*
[79] https://www.aerzteblatt.de/int/archive/article?id=127210

verbal information or suggestion. Nocebo responses may come about through unintentional negative suggestion on the part of physicians and nurses. Information about possible complications and negative expectations on the patient's part increases the likelihood of adverse effects. Adverse events under treatment with medications sometimes come about by a nocebo effect.

The above, somewhat aseptic description does not convey the severity of the problem. Although the concept has started to surface more often in recent years, we do not see the medical profession taking it as seriously as it should.

Tension Myositis Syndrome

A greatly relevant example of nocebo is given by Dr. John Sarno[80] in his book dealing with Tension Myositis Syndrome (TMS), a widespread psychosomatic condition:[81]

The pain epidemic that plagues Western society today is almost entirely a result of the nocebo. You have an attack of back and leg pain, visit the doctor and are told that it is probably a problem with the spine, most likely a herniated disc. Though TMS is harmless, being told that the pain is the direct result of a structural problem ensures that the pain will continue. Advised to stay in bed, you believe it must be serious, and the pain worsens. Despite bed rest the pain continues and an MRI is ordered; not only does it show a herniated disc at L5–S1, but the doctor informs you that the two discs above the herniated one are degenerated and the vertebral bodies are rubbing together. This is terrible; you now have objective evidence that you have

---

[80] Sarno, John E. *The Mindbody Prescription: Healing the Body, Healing the Pain.*

[81] Sarno's theory regarding the origin of TMS is not universally accepted, and alternative reasons for the condition have been offered, although the positive results he has accomplished in many cases are indisputable.

a "bad" back. Often immediate surgery is recommended, or you are told it may be necessary if you do not respond to conservative treatment. The result: intensifying pain. I have heard this history thousands of times. When finally I see the patients, they have tried every known treatment, or have had surgery, sometimes twice, for the nocebo effect has been nurtured throughout. Regardless of the treatment employed, it is always based on structural or muscle deficiency pathology, which deepens your fear and enhances the persistence of pain. Is it any wonder that some people can get better reading a book that explains the true reason for the pain and tells them that in reality they have normal backs, that most herniated discs are normal abnormalities? That is reversing the nocebo, not by placebo, but by enlisting the power of the mind to heal the body. More specifically, TMS is "cured" by teaching people to be aware of the nature of the mind–body connection.

An Old Problem, Swept Under the Rug

Nocebo is as old as human memory and has been put to negative use, for instance in societies that believe in so-called "Voodoo Death." Walter Bradford Cannon[82] reported instances of "death by fear" and other examples of nocebo already in 1942. Though much of Cannon's work was more anecdotal than clinical, his main findings are confirmed by modern science, which accounts for[83] *"the possible causes of voodoo death the role of hypothalamic CRH released after signals from the amygdala, the brain's fear center, reached the hypothalamus"* as well as the massive release of both adrenaline-like nerve chemicals and stress hormones that *"might well cause illness, including loss of appetite, weakness,*

---

[82] https://www.ncbi.nlm.nih.gov/pmc/articles/PMC1447285/pdf/0921593.pdf
[83] https://www.ncbi.nlm.nih.gov/pmc/articles/PMC1447278/pdf/0921564.pdf

cardiac arrhythmias, and even vascular collapse that could result in death."

While doctors feel the need to give realistic diagnoses to the patient, they have to take into account that their diagnosis can be wrong and that they may be creating a nocebo effect that could culminate in a self-fulfilling prophecy. Cases in which terminally ill people have miraculously healed are rare, but not unheard of, and in most cases you will find that the patients have kept their faith in the possibility of getting better, against their doctors' opinion.

Those few anecdotal incidents are the ones that we hear about, but there are countless cases in which things go differently than predicted by the treating physician, in a more modest—but still important—way. People heal without surgery and get better much sooner than predicted, and if you check those cases you will see that almost always the patient has his or her own strong assessment of the situation and does not take the doctor's predictions at face value. The importance of hope and optimism to health outcomes has been extensively researched, for instance as reported in a 2016 review published in Cureus:[84]

The optimistic attitude inherent in hopeful individuals plays a key role in successfully coping with a medical illness and its prognosis, as well as in improving health-related quality of life. This is likely due to the strong relationship between hope, resilience, and mood. Many studies have shown that mood states have a direct impact on physical health. For instance, indices of positive mood are associated with biological health markers, such as immune system response, cortisol profiles, and cardiovascular function. In contrast, negative emotional states tend to correlate with excessive somatic symptoms ... optimism predicted less probability of mortality in general and, in

---

[84] https://www.cureus.com/articles/4924-the-impact-of-hope-and-resilience-on-multiple-factors-in-neurosurgical-patients

particular, of cardiovascular mortality in a population of older adults. A study conducted on an oncological population found that low levels of hope significantly predicted premature mortality in young patients with breast cancer. Hopeful and optimistic patients with head and neck cancer showed greater survival rates a year after diagnosis when compared to pessimists ... The aforementioned studies suggest that the relationship between hope, resilience, and mood may influence physical health by encouraging involvement in health-promoting behaviors.

So when a physician gives you a diagnosis that conveys the message that "you are not going to get better," regardless of the form in which it is served to you (often in terms of percentages, as discussed before), he is doing a great disservice to you. Hope and optimism are antidotes to nocebo, and **one of the purposes of this book is to allow you realistically to distrust nocebo created by your doctor, so as to empower you to be therapeutically optimistic about the outcome of your treatment or condition, when circumstances warrant it.**

The "You Shouldn't Try That" Tribe

But nocebo doesn't harm us "only" by adversely affecting the function of our body (e.g., by having a negative effect on biological health markers, such as immune system response, cortisol profiles, and cardiovascular function). It may also have a direct and practical negative effect, when the physician discourages you from attempting a treatment that "is unlikely to help you." I gave one example in Chapter 2, when I related how a renowned professor wanted to convince me that my father's condition was hopeless and he should not attempt surgery, which he did in spite of his advice, ending up living 24 years longer than predicted to him. Taking away your hope of a solution is not an unusual event, particularly if the potentially useful therapy is considered by the medical profession to be "unscientific." The following is another, lighter but nonetheless enlightening example.

My at-the-time fifteen-year-old son got a viral wart on the plantar of his foot, which hurt like hell. We went to a dermatologist who took five seconds to remove the wart by freezing it with liquid nitrogen, and then sent us home smiling. The wart peeled off but after a short time came back again. And again. My son was miserable and the dermatologist who had treated him offered no hope, because he told us that it is a well-known fact that viral warts can keep coming back and, therefore, we should come back again for liquid nitrogen if the wart reappeared. After the third unsuccessful attempt to get rid of the wart I reminded myself that Albert Einstein defined insanity as *"doing the same thing over and over and expecting different results."* Therefore, I called an old friend of mine, a professor of dermatology, and asked his advice. He was a special person, unconventional, open-minded, and widely knowledgeable, and I trusted that if anybody knew how to help, he would.

"You should try guided imagery," he said.

"Try guided what?!" I asked.

"That is an effective way to get rid of recurrent viral warts," he explained patiently. "It works."

I didn't place much hope in the suggested witchcraft, but for want of a better idea I contacted the physician that my friend had recommended and took my son to see him. He sat down with my son for three half-hour sessions, made him imagine that he was walking on hot sand at the beach, and, using only words, healed him of the persistent wart.

My friend and the treating physician seemed to view it as a routine treatment, but to me it was mind-boggling. Did guided imagery work only for specific conditions, such as viral warts, I asked myself, or had it a more universal effect? And what were the limits of the control that our mind has over our body? I have since learned that our mind has a much greater power over our body than we realize. I have also learned that most physicians will either not know or believe that alternative treatments may help in some cases, or may be afraid to be labeled as quacks if they suggest one. In spite of the fact that this treatment is very well documented in the medical literature,[85] it took someone like my friend, with his professional self-assurance and broad knowledge and understanding of our body, to suggest such an "outlandish" solution to the trivial problem of a recurring viral wart. Whether the dermatologist who treated my son was not aware of this option, or knew about it but didn't feel like suggesting it after the second unsuccessful attempt to get rid of the wart, doesn't really matter. It only shows you, once again, that when you have a medical problem, much of the time you are really on your own.

Takeaways from This Chapter:

▶ The term "Nocebo" refers to an effect opposite to that of placebo (in which a sugar pill cures a condition). It may be brought about by a physician who unwittingly conveys to a patient a wrong image of his condition.

▶ A host of conditions (such as Tension Myositis Syndrome) may be psychosomatic in origin. A wrong attitude of a treating physician may make them worse.

▶ Your doctor may discourage you from attempting a certain therapy because (at least to him) it is unconventional. Before accepting his conclusion, you must make up your mind on the basis of actual, reliable and published data. Unsurprisingly, your doctor may be wrong.

[85] https://www.ncbi.nlm.nih.gov/pmc/articles/PMC3218765/pdf/prbm-3-051.pdf

CHAPTER 11
Your Survival Kit

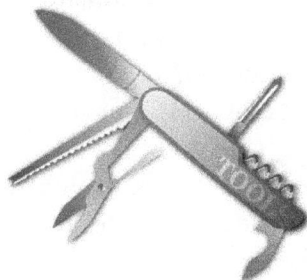

I call the following suggestions "Survival Kit," because any one of them may help you to gain a better understanding of the circumstances surrounding your condition and the treatment offered to you. It will point out to you some tools that you may use to increase your knowledge and understanding of your situation, and a better understanding means an increased chance that you will make right decisions and get the appropriate treatment. It is of course impossible to translate into a structured procedure what should be the proper way to act when we receive a diagnosis. That would be tantamount to offering "a protocol," which we know may sometimes be a misleading and harmful way to go. However, I have listed below in concentrated form some suggestions for action. These summarize the conclusions from what was discussed in this book, regarding matters that you should take into account in various situations.

I know that after reading the checklists below you will say that this is a lot of work for you to undertake in a field in which you feel uncertain and may have no prior knowledge or understanding about whatsoever. Starting clueless in a completely foreign field may be daunting. But do you have anything more important to do than making sure that you are getting the right and best treatment? If you are busy with more important things, then you can put yourself blindly in the hands of your doctor, delegate your health to the medical system, shut your eyes to the facts, and hope for the best. After all, Life is a gamble.

A. Upon receipt of a diagnosis, consider these questions:
1. How well does your doctor know you, your medical history, and your general condition?
2. Does he come across as empathetic, or impatient or disinterested?
3. Doctors often speak in terms of likelihood. How "likely" does your doctor think that the tests are conclusive?
4. How well does the diagnosis fit with your body's feelings? Is there anything in the diagnosis that clashes with what your body is telling you? (See Chapter 3.)
5. Are there any other tests that could support the diagnosis, which have not been run because your doctor doesn't feel that they are needed "in your case" (or cost more money and your health provider will not allow you to take them unless specific circumstances warrant it)?
6. How common and widespread is the diagnosed condition? For instance, if it is a seasonal illness (such as, for instance, the flu in winter), could it be that your doctor is too quick to group you with other patients showing similar symptoms? (See Chapter 4 for WYSIATI.)

7. Is the diagnosed condition within the field in which your doctor specializes?[86] If so, before taking potentially unnecessary tests, it might be wise to consult with someone knowledgeable in that specific field.
8. If the conclusion is that nothing is wrong with you, is there any other clear and reasonable explanation for the events that brought you to the doctor? If one is offered, is there any test that can validate it that has not been prescribed?
9. Taking all the above considerations into account together, how confident do you feel about your doctor's diagnosis on an intuitive level?

10. Before accepting the diagnosis, consider doing the following:

a. Do your own research, keeping the answers to all the above questions in mind, to find **recent** literature focused on your condition, for instance, by researching the PubMed Central database[87] (US National Library of Medicine National Institutes of Health)—see also below. Medical findings change with time as new information is added and Big Data is analyzed, so please refer to the most up-to-date results (although important information can also be found in earlier work). You want to know as much as possible about the condition and its treatment, but from reliable sources, not only from anecdotal posts by other patients. This knowledge may be helpful to the success of the treatment and may also help you to find clues to a potentially wrong diagnosis or a mistreatment.

b. Read the articles, concentrating on the diagnostic conclusions (you will return to those articles later, when considering treatment). Much of it may be gibberish to you at first and you

---

[86] If your symptoms fit a condition outside his field of expertise, you may become the subject of unnecessary testing to satisfy the doctor's insecurity.
[87] https://www.ncbi.nlm.nih.gov/pmc

may need the help of someone with knowledge in the field to fully understand it, but a first reading may raise some red flags for you, which may help you to inquire deeper. For instance, if most patients with your supposed condition have low vitamin D and your levels are perfect, your doctor will have to convince you why this does not put a question mark against his diagnosis. It may very well be that he is still right, but you want to have the specific answer to that question.

c. If your research brings up information that was not considered by your physician or that he did not discuss with you, discuss it with him and obtain clear answers to any question that has arisen. Do not be shy about demanding answers and do not let your doctor evade questions. Don't feel bad about bringing him relevant articles you have found and ignore his rolling eyes. This is about your health and you must take control of it as much as you can.

◆

B. Before starting treatment consider these points:
1. If the proposed treatment is not something conventional (like an antibiotic for an infection), try to find out if your doctor is engaged in research, or whether he is taking part in a clinical trial somehow related to the treatment, or is in any way connected to the treatment other than by way of prescribing it for his patients. You may make some tactful inquiries with him, or see possible courses of action below.
2. Find out what the alternative treatments available for your condition are.
3. Determine how long the treatment has been used and what the results are **in numbers**. Remember: Never take an answer in percentages. If your doctor tells you that the treatment was successful in 80% of the cases, it may mean that 160,000 people out of 200,000 have had success with it, which indicates that the treatment is generally good (but not necessarily that it is

good for your particular situation), but it can also mean that 8 people out of 10, who have so far tried it, have been successful, which is meaningless.

4. Make sure to understand the side effects of the treatment and the potential dangers. If the chances of a side effect are tiny, but the potential negative outcome is catastrophic, you may want to consider alternative therapy.

5. Then consider doing the following:

a. You need to know whether your doctor is partial to a certain treatment because he has a personal interest in it that may affect his judgment in respect of your condition. If he didn't volunteer that information, you may want to check out:

1) Whether he is taking part in a clinical trial involving the procedure or one of the drugs he is prescribing, or has done so in the past. You can easily find that information through the https://clinicaltrials.gov database. Simply enter your doctor's name in the "Other terms" field:

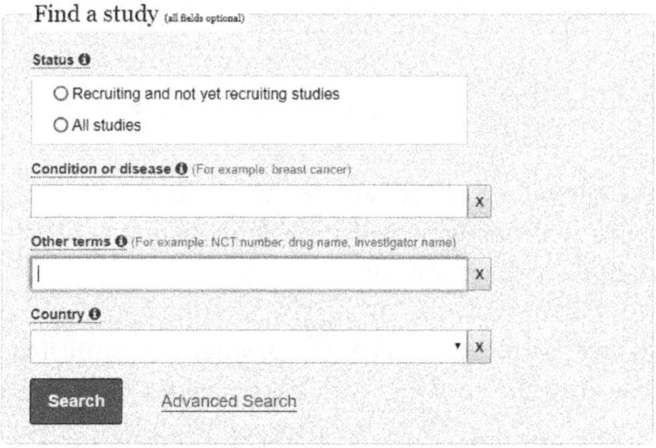

Find a study (all fields optional)

Status ❶
- ○ Recruiting and not yet recruiting studies
- ○ All studies

Condition or disease ❶ (For example: breast cancer)

Other terms ❶ (For example: NCT number, drug name, investigator name)

Country ❶

Search   Advanced Search

Fig. 5: Search form from https://clinicaltrials.gov

The result will be a list of clinical trials that will tell you if your doctor is involved in researching anything relating to your condition. You can narrow down the results by including the condition or disease in the search terms. This is a quite simple way to find information relevant to your situation.

2) Whether he is doing research (other than clinical trials) on a subject related to your condition. This is important because his judgement may be affected by the aims of his research and his personal expectations. To do that you need to go to the advanced search screen of PubMed at https://www.ncbi.nlm.nih.gov/pubmed/advanced and select "Author" as the first field, in which you will write your doctor's name:

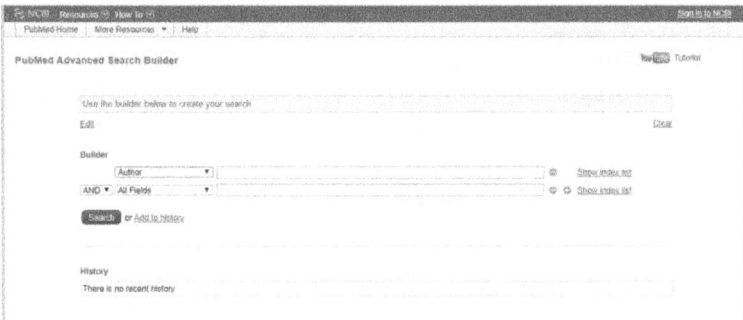

Fig. 6: Advanced Search Page in PubMed

The result will be a list of articles in which your doctor appears as an author, and you will be able to pick any article that is relevant to your condition.

b. Read any article that has come up, whether connected to your doctor or not, looking for discrepancies that need to be reconciled. For instance, if the paper says that among the patients who did not respond well to the treatment, 30% were medicated for high blood pressure, and you are taking blood pressure medication, you must ask your doctor what that means for you. He may have overlooked that particular angle, but you won't overlook it because it is all about you and you couldn't care more.

◆

C. Before agreeing to surgery, consider these points:

1. Surgery is often proposed as the right solution to a problem, while alternative solutions, such as physical therapy, exist, which do not require cutting into your body. (See Chapter 8.) Surgeons seldom suggest physical therapy or medication, because that's not what they are trained to do.

2. The risks of surgery are often underplayed and because you want to get rid of the pain that has been making you miserable, the vision of a simple and quick solution triggers your "It Will Not Happen to Me" response. You need to resist it and to make a decision with all the facts in hand.

3. Consider doing the following:

a. Research your condition, available treatments, and risks, as in (B) above.

b. Use the ACS Risk Calculator **to ask your surgeon questions, not to reach conclusions**. This calculator,[88] provided by the American College of Surgeons, is in principle intended for the use of surgeons, not of patients. It allows inputting your health data and on that basis it calculates various risks connected with the planned surgery. Fig. 7 below shows the results of the risk calculator for an overweight male aged 65–74, who takes medication for diabetes and hypertension and is considering spinal fusion surgery.

If we glance at the results superficially, it all looks good. Negative outcome appears to be mostly below average and we are not predicted to stay at the hospital for more than 2.5 days. But let's now look at these results a bit more closely. After those 2.5 days we have a 10.6% chance that we won't be allowed to go home. Instead, we may have to be admitted to a nursing or

---

[88] https://riskcalculator.facs.org/RiskCalculator

rehab facility. This means that 11 out of every 100 patients of the same type will not go home after surgery.

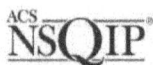

ACS NSQIP | Surgical Risk Calculator

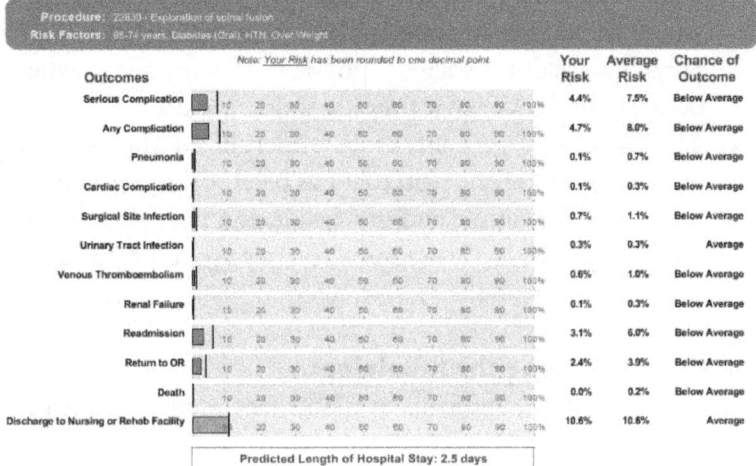

Fig. 7: Surgical Risk Calculator Results

Looking at the scale, we may feel reassured to see that we have a "below average" chance (4.4%) of serious complications. A closer look, however, will tell us that this means that 5 patients out of 100 are likely to suffer one or more of the following important problems that occur after surgery, including:
• Heart complication: Includes heart attack or sudden stopping of the heart
• Pneumonia: Infection in the lungs
• Kidney failure: Kidneys no longer function in making urine and/or clearing the blood of toxins
• Blood clot: Clot in the legs or lungs
• Return to the OR: The need to go back to the operating room due to a problem after the prior surgery

• Wound infection: An infection at or near the area where the surgery was performed
• Sepsis: Whole-body infection
• Intubation: The need to put the breathing tube back in after surgery to help breathing
• Urinary tract infection: Infection of the bladder and kidneys
• Wound disruption: Separation of the layers of a surgical wound

But that's not all that we can expect. We also have a 4.7% chance of "any complication," which includes:
• Wound infection: An infection at or near the incision
• Extended time on the ventilator: Ventilator assistance for breathing longer than 48 hours
• Stroke: An interruption in blood flow to the brain

When we put it like that, one must be out of his mind to undergo this surgery as long as alternative, non-surgical options exist. But unless you spend time exploring the meaning of what is planned for you, internalize it, and discuss it in detail with your surgeon, you may be swayed by beautiful graphs that show you how below average your chances of an adverse outcome are.

Takeaways from This Chapter:

► Knowledge is power. You want to learn as much as possible about your condition and its treatment.
► You have access to the information that you need to be able to get answers to important questions from your health providers. Learn to use those sources.
► Statistics often look better than they in fact are. Always humanize them by looking at their meaning for you.

> ▶ Always demand explanations of the meaning of generic terms like "complications" to understand what they may mean to you and to your future life, before agreeing to take unnecessary risks.

CHAPTER 12
Final Words

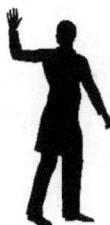

Before We Go

This book could have been written by you and by many other people who have lost their faith in the ability of the medical system to manage their health problem without their help. I have not discovered any secret information. Throughout this book you won't find anything that is not freely available to everybody who has the will to search and read. Amazingly, however, efforts to take all the avalanche of information that hits the web on a daily basis, distill it, and turn it into a humanly understandable picture, are few and far between. That's why I have taken it upon myself to do this job.

It is very important to me that the message coming from this book not be misunderstood as meaning that the medical system is worthless and that the advice of physicians should be ignored. The medical system brings us huge achievements that extend our life and its quality. It has one central flaw, however: it does not function uniformly well unless the patient exercises vigilance over the solutions that the system is capable of providing him or her. Like in other systems that have grown large, complex, and elitist, the underlying assumption is that the patient cannot understand much or contribute a lot and that the doctor knows better. While that may be true in some cases, it is not a general truth. In order to illustrate that point I had to bring up troubling examples, because bad doctors and even crooked ones exist and we, the patients, have no easy means of telling who they are, unless we put in the effort to question, learn, and argue as needed.

I think that the appropriate way to end this book is by repeating what I already said in Chapter 1: that many and possibly most doctors are great persons, who do their best to help us when we need them. Unfortunately, limitations imposed on them by the system, budgets, and demands on their time often make their job difficult if not impossible. We sympathize with their problems, but we must first look after our own, because we don't have the luxury to be understanding when dealing with mistakes that may harm our health and that of our family.

I hope that the takeaway from this book is that we shouldn't rely on luck when dealing with our health and, instead, we should strive to learn and understand everything we can. Having said that, however, and since it never hurts, I wish you good luck too!

Meet the Author:

Kfir Luzzatto is the author of eleven novels, several short stories, and six non-fiction books. Kfir was born and raised in Italy, and moved to Israel as a teenager. He acquired the love for the English language from his father, a former U.S. soldier, a voracious reader, and a prolific writer. Kfir has a PhD in chemical engineering and works as a patent attorney. He lives in Omer, Israel, with his full-time partner, Esther, their four children, Michal, Lilach, Tamar, and Yonatan, and the dog Elvis.

In pursuit of his interest in the mind-body connection, Kfir was certified as a Clinical Hypnotherapist by the Anglo European College of Therapeutic Hypnosis.

Kfir has published extensively in the professional and general press over the years. For almost four years he wrote a weekly "Patents" column in Globes (Israel's financial newspaper). His popular guide, *FUN WITH PATENTS—The Irreverent Guide for the Investor, the Entrepreneur and the Inventor*, was published in 2016. He is an HWA (Horror Writers Association) and ITW (International Thriller Writers) member.

Kfir's mind–body website is www.DoItWithWords.com and you can also visit his literary website at www.KfirLuzzatto.com.

Follow him on Twitter (@KfirLuzzatto) and on Facebook: https://www.facebook.com/KfirLuzzattoAuthor.

Appendix 1
Cover of "The American Frugal Housewife"

THE

AMERICAN

FRUGAL HOUSEWIFE.

DEDICATED TO THOSE

WHO ARE NOT ASHAMED OF ECONOMY.

BY MRS. CHILD,

AUTHOR OF "HOBOMOK," "THE MOTHER'S BOOK," EDITOR OF THE
"JUVENILE MISCELLANY," &c.

A fat kitchen maketh a lean will.—FRANKLIN.

"Economy is a poor man's revenue; extravagance a rich man's ruin.

TWELFTH EDITION.
ENLARGED AND CORRECTED BY THE AUTHOR.

BOSTON:
CARTER, HENDEE, AND CO.
1833.

Appendix 2
Cover of "The Cottage Physician"

THE
Cottage Physician

FOR INDIVIDUAL AND FAMILY USE.

PREVENTION, SYMPTOMS AND TREATMENT.

BEST KNOWN METHODS

IN ALL

Diseases, Accidents and Emergencies of the Home.

PREPARED BY

The Best Physicians and Surgeons of Modern Practice.

ALLOPATHY, + HOMŒOPATHY,

ETC., ETC.

WITH INTRODUCTION BY

GEORGE W. POST, A.M., M.D.,

Adjunct

Professor of the Practice of Medicine

IN THE

COLLEGE OF PHYSICIANS AND SURGEONS, CHICAGO.

Complete Hand Book of Medical Knowledge for the Home.

NEARLY 200 ILLUSTRATIONS.

The King-Richardson Co.

Springfield, Mass.

RICHMOND.   DES MOINES.   INDIANAPOLIS.   SAN JOSÉ.
DALLAS.   1900   TOLEDO.

. 119 .